6.80

Interferon 1980

Interferon 1980

Volume 2

ION GRESSER
Editor-in-chief

1980

ACADEMIC PRESS
A Subsidiary of Harcourt Brace Jovanovich, Publishers
London New York Toronto Sydney
San Francisco

ACADEMIC PRESS INC. (LONDON) LTD.
24/28 Oval Road,
London NW1

United States Edition published by
ACADEMIC PRESS INC.
111 Fifth Avenue
New York, New York 10003

British Library Cataloguing in Publication Data
Interferon.
Vol. 2: 1980
1. Interferons
I. Gresser, Ion
612′.0157′5 QR187.5 79–41412
ISBN 0–12–302251–7

Text set in 10/12pt Monophoto Times New Roman

Filmset by Northumberland Press Ltd,
Gateshead, Tyne and Wear
Printed in Great Britain by
Fletcher & Son Ltd, Norwich

Contributors

P. E. Bigazzi, *Department of Pathology, University of Connecticut Health Center, Farmington, Connecticut 06032, USA*

D. C. Burke, *Department of Biological Sciences, University of Warwick, Coventry CV4 7AL, UK*

S. Cohen, *Department of Pathology, University of Connecticut Health Center, Farmington, Connecticut 06032, USA*

Committee on Interferon Nomenclature, *Interferon Laboratories, Memorial Sloan-Kettering Cancer Center, 1275 New York Avenue, New York, New York 10021, USA*

N. B. Finter, *Wellcome Research Laboratories, Langley Court, Beckenham, Kent BR3 3BS, UK*

K. H. Fantes, *Wellcome Research Laboratories, Langley Court, Beckenham, Kent BR3 3BS, UK*

E. Knight, Jr, *Central Research and Development Department, E. I. Du Pont de Nemours and Company, Wilmington, Delaware, USA*

J. Taylor-Papadimitriou, *Imperial Cancer Research Fund, PO Box 123, Lincoln's Inn Fields, London WC2A 3PX, UK*

Contents

The Type I Human Interferon Gene System; Chromosomal Location and Control of Gene Expression

Derek C. Burke

The Purity and Safety of Interferons Prepared for Clinical Use: The Case for Lymphoblastoid Interferon

N. B. Finter and K. H. Fantes

Lymphokines, Cytokines and Interferon(s)

Stanley Cohen and Pierluigi E. Bigazzi

Purification and Characterization of Interferons

ERNEST KNIGHT, Jr

Central Research and Development Department, E. I. Du Pont de Nemours, Wilmington, Delaware, USA

I INTRODUCTION

The best way to describe the progress in purification and characterization of the interferon proteins is that it has just begun. As in the study of other biological molecules and in the pursuance of religion, purity must precede understanding. Moreover, characterizing an interferon before it is pure is like characterizing a child before it is born, some things may change. The purification to homogeneity and characterization, beyond generalities, of the interferons has been a long and tortuous journey. However, considerable progress has been made in the last few years and it should accelerate in the future.

The purpose of this article is two-fold: (1) the presentation of some facts, opinions (biased), and speculations on the purification and characterization of those interferons that have been obtained pure; (2) the description of some experiences and interactions with other scientists in the pursuit of pure interferon during the past decade. In some cases where personal comments are used, names will be omitted to protect the innocent (and my personal safety). This article is not intended to be a thorough review of the literature on this subject. Reviews are available and the reader is recommended to them for a more comprehensive survey (Stewart, 1979a). My intent is to review only those interferons that have been obtained pure and to compare and evaluate their chemical and biological properties. The purification procedures for obtaining pure interferons are varied and ingeneous and the reader is referred to the original publications for details.

II PURIFICATION OF INTERFERONS

> Pure is: (1) having a homogeneous or uniform composition, not mixed: (2) free from adulterants or impurities; full-strength: (3) free from dirt, defilement, or pollution; clean: (4) free from foreign elements: (5) containing nothing inappropriate or extraneous.
>
> The American Heritage Dictionary of the English Language

> For our knowledge is imperfect and our prophecy is imperfect; but when the perfect comes, the imperfect will pass away.
>
> St Paul, First Corinthians 14:9, 10

The discoverers and early workers with interferon realized the necessity to obtain pure interferon. Little did they know of the long and arduous task ahead to obtain the minute quantities of the pure interferons that we have today. Why has it been difficult to obtain pure interferons? First, the biological activity of an interferon is extremely potent (effective at 10^{-12}–10^{-13} M on cells in culture). A cell does not make very much, thus there is very little starting material. Second, it is an inducible system and not a constitutive one; therefore it has to be obtained from animals or cells growing in culture since the usual sources of polypeptide hormones, animal organs, contain no interferon. Clearly there is no chance of obtaining sufficient quantities of a pure interferon if there is insufficient starting material. Third, there is the assay; it is slow and imprecise. Very few scientists will undertake the purification of a protein whose assay requires 2–3 days. For example, a purification step may be performed and if the interferon is unstable, the activity may disappear by the time the results of the assay are obtained. Thus it is possible not to get beyond the first step in a purification since most of the interferon may be lost by the time its activity is determined.

Although the word interferon is often used in the singular (*Time Magazine*, 1980) there is more than one protein with interferon activity. The early research on interferon indicated some species specificity, suggesting that all interferons are not the same protein. The first attempts to purify an interferon were with chick interferon, the system where interferon was discovered. In 1967, Karl Fantes and I. G. S. Furminger (Fantes and Furminger, 1967) reported results which were to foretell the future of interferon purifications for the next 10 years. After extensive purification of chick interferon they discovered that on electrophoretic analysis of the proteins and interferon activity, the activity did not reside in any detected protein! All persons who have attempted to purify an interferon have experienced the same result, activity but no identifiable protein. Such results have sent the experimenters into the depths of depression and have caused them to consider other lines of work. After I had had a similar experience someone said to me, "Well, maybe we will never characterize or understand an interferon". Other indignities have been suffered. Comments such as "I believe you have extensively purified the interferon but that band on the gel isn't really interferon", were received with sullen resignation. However, in spite of painfully slow progress, and pessimistic predictions from their friends, those that purify interferons (masochists that they are) have persisted and prevailed.

Probably no one who has been involved in the purification of an interferon believed initially that it would be as difficult as it has been. Little did I know of the problems ahead when, in 1973, Ed Havell and Jan Vilček gave me some human fibroblast cells for the production of interferon. As I departed their laboratory with the cells they shook my hand and wished me luck in the purification. I did not realize at that time that the cells in the two small flasks that they gave me would later produce so many cells and so little interferon.

A further complicating factor in the purification of the interferons has been the discoveries that more than one interferon can be produced by a cell or by different cells from the same animal. There appear to be at least three mouse interferons and four human interferons (for a review of these interferons see Stewart, 1979a). Those interferons that have been obtained pure are shown in Table I. The methods of their purification have been

TABLE I Pure Human and Mouse Interferons

Type of interferon	Molecular weight	Reference
Human fibroblast	20 000	Knight (1976a, b)
Human fibroblastoid	19 000	Berthold *et al.* (1978)
Human leukocyte	18 000	Rubinstein *et al.* (1979)
Human leukocyte	18 400–22 100 (5 proteins)	Berg and Heron (1980a)
Human lymphoblastoid	18 500	Zoon *et al.* (1979)
Mouse L cell	22 000–38 000 (9–10 proteins)	Knight (1975)
Mouse C-243 cells	22 000, 35 000 (2 proteins)	De Maeyer-Guignard *et al.* (1978)
Mouse L cells	24 000, 40 000 (2 proteins)	Iwakura *et al.* (1978)
Mouse Ehrlich ascites tumour cells	35 000, 26 000, 20 000 (3 proteins—A, B, C)	Kawakita *et al.* (1978)

omitted but the details are available in the references listed. All the recent purifications have focused on the human and mouse interferons. These interferons have held the most scientific interest and cell culture methods for their production have been developed. The reader should be aware that those pure interferons listed have been obtained only in microgram quantities.

However, the old question returns. How do you know it is pure? How can you be sure that the protein you are analysing is *really* interferon? These are tiresome but appropriate questions. First, those interferons listed in Table I migrate as one protein band coincident with the biological activity when subjected to electrophoresis in polyacrylamide gels containing sodium dodecyl sulphate. This is a widely accepted method for determining the purity of a protein. Second, all have been purified to similar final specific activities. In my opinion, arguments about specific activities and absolute purity are futile, given the unavoidable imprecision and inaccuracy in making the measurements for specific activity calculations. (Once at a scientific meeting a friend said that he believed that the specific activity of pure interferon was about 10^{11} units/mg. I am eternally thankful that he was not right or we would now have nanograms of pure interferons instead of micrograms). Third, *N*-terminal amino acid sequences of some human and mouse interferons have been obtained. The data show that there is, in each case, only one protein in the preparation (i.e. only one sequence of amino acids). Thus, I believe it has been demonstrated beyond doubt that both human and mouse interferons have been obtained pure, albeit in very small amounts. On the other hand, a die-hard sceptic might say that an inert protein has been isolated with physical properties very similar to the interferon and that coincidentally the interferon activity purifies with it (in other words, the ultimate specific activity really is 10^{11} units/mg).

III CHARACTERIZATION OF INTERFERONS

Since some interferons can now be obtained pure (Table I) it is essential that chemical and physical properties be characterized. Furthermore, since the discovery of interferon, numerous nonantiviral effects have been attributed to the interferons albeit mostly with interferons in impure preparations (Stewart, 1979b). As with the chemical and physical properties it is also essential to determine which biologic effects attributed to interferons in impure preparations can be demonstrated with pure interferons. I will briefly review and comment first on the chemical and physical properties of the pure interferons and second on the biologic effects caused by the pure interferons.

A Chemical and Physical Properties of Pure Interferons

The only physical property of the pure interferons that has been determined is their molecular weights (shown in Table I). They have been calculated from mobilities observed after electrophoresis in polyacrylamide gels containing sodium dodecylsulphate. These molecular weights are probably not an accurate reflection of amino acid composition since interferons are glycoproteins containing an unknown amount of carbohydrate. The molecular weight of one human leukocyte interferon has been calculated from the amino acid composition (Rubinstein *et al.*, 1979) and that of human lymphoblastoid interferon has been obtained (by electrophoresis) after extensive deglycosylation of the interferon (Zoon *et al.*, 1979). The molecular weights of the human interferons cluster in the range 15 000–25 000. The pure mouse interferons range from 22 000 to 38 000 (Table I). As mentioned earlier, a complication in the purification of some of the interferons has been their size heterogeneity. For instance one group (Rubinstein *et al.*, 1979) purified one leukocyte interferon to homogeneity, but their purification procedure (high performance liquid chromatography) revealed the existence of other leukocyte interferons. Another group purified five leukocyte interferons to homogeneity (Berg and Heron, 1980a). The relationships among these leukocyte interferons that have been purified by different procedures is not clear and further work must be done to clarify them. Human fibroblast and human fibroblastoid interferons have been obtained pure (Table I) from diploid fibroblasts and transformed fibroblasts respectively and recent experiments (Okamura *et al.*, 1980) indicate that they may be identical proteins.

The pure mouse interferons show considerable size heterogeneity. One report (Knight, 1975) stated that 9–10 interferons could be obtained pure. These interferons were obtained from mouse cells induced by MM virus. Other pure mouse interferons have been obtained from mouse C-243 cells (De Maeyer-Guignard *et al.*, 1978), mouse L cells (Iwakura *et al.*, 1978) and mouse Ehrlich ascites tumour cells (Kawakita *et al.* 1978); the inducer in each case was Newcastle disease virus (NDV). All three cell lines produced two or three interferons when purified to homogeneity (Table I). Why mouse L cells induced with MM virus should produce more interferons than other mouse cells induced by NDV is not clear at present. We will have to wait on the answer to this question as no one, to my knowledge, is using MM virus as an inducer for the large scale preparation of interferon (Knight became interested in human interferon). All characterization of mouse interferons is being done with interferons produced by NDV-induced cells.

The identity (or lack of identity) of human fibroblast, fibroblastoid, leukocyte and lymphoblastoid interferons in amino acid sequence has been the subject of considerable speculation. It has been suggested that some of the differences in physical (molecular weights) and chemical (antibody cross reactivity) properties could be the result solely of differences in carbohydrate content rather than differences in amino acid sequence. The amino acid composition has been determined for one human leukocyte interferon (Rubinstein *et al.*, 1979), human lymphoblastoid interferon (Zoon *et al.*, 1979), human fibroblastoid interferon (Tan *et al.*, 1979) and human fibroblast interferon (Knight *et al.*, 1980). There are significant differences in the amino acid compositions indicating different amino acid sequences. Furthermore, amino acid sequences at the *N*-terminal of human fibroblast (Knight *et al.*, 1980) and human lymphoblastoid (Zoon *et al.*, 1980) interferon have been determined (Table II). The *N*-terminal sequences of the two interferons are different, therefore they are different proteins.

First, the *N*-terminal amino acid sequencing and how it was performed. When scientists that sequence proteins by standard methods are asked how much protein they need to begin their experiments, they respond by saying 1 mg, minimum. This is a very modest request to them but 1 mg of pure interferon still boggles the minds of those that purify interferons. In 1978, however, the development at the California Institute of Technology of methods for obtaining substantial amino acid sequence on sub-nanomole quantities of a protein was reported (Hunkapiller and Hood, 1978; 1980). This technology seemed ideally suited for the sequencing of interferons and collaborations were established between the California Institute of Technology and groups that had small amounts of pure interferons. These collaborations led to publication in February, 1980 of the *N*-terminal sequences of human fibroblast and human lymphoblastoid interferons and two mouse interferons. Table II shows a comparison of *N*-terminal sequences of these interferons. It is clear that human fibroblast and lymphoblastoid interferons are not identical proteins since there is only one homologous amino acid (leucine at position 9) in the first 13 residues. Recent experiments show that the first 13 amino acids at the *N*-terminal of human fibroblastoid interferon (Okamura *et al.*, 1980) have the same sequence as those at the *N*-terminal of human fibroblast interferon (Table II). This *N*-terminal homology suggests that they are the same proteins, but further sequence must be obtained from both to prove it. In the first 20 *N*-terminal residues of the mouse interferons there is homology at only two positions (glutamine at 5 and lysine at 16) thus proving that they are different proteins. This conclusion had been suggested earlier by tryptic mapping of the two mouse interferons (Iwakura *et al.*, 1978; Cabrer *et al.*, 1979). The homology that was the least expected was that between the human and mouse interferons (Table II). Thirteen of the 20 amino acids at the *N*-terminal of human lymphoblastoid and mouse C interferons are identical while three of 13 of human fibroblast and mouse A interferons are identical. What these homologies mean for biological activity or for evolution we cannot even speculate but what is

TABLE II *N*-Terminal Amino Acid Sequences of Human and Mouse Interferons

Interferon	*n*-Terminal sequence	References
Human fibroblast	H-Met-Ser-Tyr-Asn-[5]Leu-Leu-Gly-Phe-Leu-[10]Gln-Arg-Ser-Ser	Knight *et al.* (1980)
Human lymphoblastoid	H-Ser-Asp-Leu-Pro-Gln-Thr-His-Ser-Leu-Gly-Asn-Arg-Arg-[15]Ala-Leu-Ile-Leu-Leu-Ala-[20]Gln	Zoon *et al.* (1980)
Mouse A and B	H-Ile-Asn-Tyr-Lys-Gln-Leu-Gln-Leu-Gln-Glu-Arg-Thr-Asn-Ile-Arg-Lys-?-Gln-Glu-Leu-Leu-Glu-Gln-Leu	Taira *et al.* (1980)
Mouse C	H-Ala-Asp-Leu-Pro-Gln-Thr-Tyr-Asn-Leu-Gly-Asn-Lys-Gly-Ala-Leu-Lys-Val-Leu-Ala-Gln	Taira *et al.* (1980)
Human fibroblast	H-Met-Ser-Tyr-Asn-Leu-Leu-Gly-Phe-Leu-Gln-Arg-Ser-Ser	
Mouse A and B	H-Ile-Asn-Tyr-Lys-Gln-Leu-Gln-Leu-Gln-Glu-Arg-Thr-Asn	
Human lymphoblastoid	H-Ser-Asp-Leu-Pro-Gln-Thr-His-Ser-Leu-Gly-Asn-Arg-Arg-Ala-Leu-Ile-Leu-Leu-Ala-Gln	
Mouse C	H-Ala-Asp-Leu-Pro-Gln-Thr-Tyr-Asn-Leu-Gly-Asn-Lys-Gly-Ala-Leu-Lys-Val-Leu-Ala-Gln	

strongly suggested is that we are investigating a family of proteins. Furthermore, this demonstrates to the next to last sceptic that we really have purified and sequenced interferons. The last sceptic will not be convinced yet, but read on, there is more to come.

The use of recombinant DNA technology for the cloning of eukaryotic genes into bacteria has developed rapidly and is being widely used. Considerable publicity has been devoted in the past year to the cloning of an interferon gene. Recently, the cloning of human fibroblast (Taniguchi *et al.*, 1980a) and human leukocyte (Nagata *et al.*, 1980) interferons has been reported. The fibroblast interferon cDNA synthesized from interferon messenger RNA, was cloned into a bacterial plasmid. The DNA sequence for the fibroblast interferon in the bacterial plasmid was identified by sequencing a plasmid DNA (identified as containing a probable fibroblast gene by biological methods) and locating a DNA sequence that could be translated into the 13 amino acid sequence which had been obtained from the fibroblast protein (Table II). The gene for human leukocyte interferon was cloned in a similar manner and was identified by isolating a bacterium that produced leukocyte-like interferon activity (antiviral). The plasmid DNA of the leukocyte gene has also been sequenced (Mantei *et al.*, 1980). Its sequence when converted into amino acid sequence is homologous in 15 of 20 amino acids to the *N*-terminal sequence obtained from the lymphoblastoid interferon protein. These data show that the leukocyte and lymphoblastoid interferons are very similar at their *N*-terminals. In both fibroblast (Taniguchi *et al.*, 1980a) and leukocyte (Mantei *et al.*, 1980) genes the DNA sequence predicts interferon polypeptides of 166 amino acids. There are no data yet available on the amino acid sequence obtained from the leukocyte protein nor are sequence data available from the DNA of a cloned lymphoblastoid interferon. Whether the complete amino acid sequences obtained from the interferon proteins will be identical to that derived from the cloned DNAs remains to be determined.

Human fibroblast interferon DNA and human leukocyte interferon DNA have been compared (Taniguchi *et al.*, 1980b) and the authors point out that there is 45% homology at the nucleotide and 29% homology at the amino acid level. Moreover, this is a clear indication to them that these two interferons are from the same family of proteins. The identical homology between the fibroblast interferon *N*-terminal sequence obtained from the protein and that derived from the fibroblast DNA should silence the last critic, but I doubt it. At a future meeting someone may ask, "Well, do you really believe that that protein is interferon?"

Is the carbohydrate moiety of those interferons that have been obtained pure necessary for activity *in vitro*? Probably not, but a definite answer must await further experimentation. Human lymphoblastoid interferon has been extensively deglycosylated and it retains activity (Zoon *et al.*, 1979). Several interferons that have been obtained pure, human leukocyte (Rubinstein *et al.*, 1979), mouse interferon (Knight, 1975; De Maeyer-Guignard *et al.*, 1978), contain very little or no carbohydrate but yet are active *in vitro*. The results should be taken only as indications and not proof of active interferons without carbohydrate. The carbohydrate composition of an interferon may vary from preparation to preparation since a cell controls the polymerization of carbohydrates less rigidly than the polymerization of amino acids.

B Biologic Properties of Pure Interferons

The varied biologic effects of the interferons have been recently reviewed (Stewart, 1979a) and it is my intention only to point out those effects which have been shown to be caused by a pure interferon. All the pure interferons shown in Table I were purified as antiviral activities, thus it is important to ask if the pure interferons will (or will not) cause some or all of the biologic effects that have been attributed to interferon preparations. In 1976 it was reported that homogeneous human fibroblast interferon would inhibit the growth of cells in culture (Table III). It has taken 14–17 years to prove

TABLE III Inhibition of the Growth of Cells in Culture by Pure Interferons

Interferon	Cells inhibited	Reference
Human fibroblast	Human fibroblast	Knight (1976a, b)
Human leukocyte	Human lymphoblastoid	Evinger *et al.*, (1980)
Human leukocyte	Human lymphoblastoid	Berg and Heron (1980b)
Mouse	Murine leukaemia L1210	De Meyer-Guignard *et al.* (1978)
Mouse	Mouse L cells	Iwakura *et al.* (1978)

that the original observation (Paucker *et al.*, 1962) was in fact caused by interferon. There have been no exceptions, all the interferons that have been obtained pure, and have been tested, inhibit the growth of cells in culture (Table III). For those who have been associated with this area of interferon research this is a satisfying answer and conclusion to a major question.

There are other nonantiviral effects caused by interferons. Those non-antiviral effects, other than the inhibition of cell growth, that have been caused by pure interferons are shown in Table IV. These effects had been observed earlier with impure preparations of interferons and these experiments and observations have been reviewed (Stewart, 1979b). The most extensive study of non-antiviral activities has been made with pure mouse interferon (Gresser *et al.*, 1979; Table IV). Similar observations have been made with pure human leukocyte interferon (Berg and Heron, 1980c; Table

TABLE IV Nonantiviral[a] Activities of Pure Interferons

Interferon	Activity	Reference
Mouse	Inhibition of growth of a transplantable tumour in mice	Gresser *et al.* (1979)
Mouse	Enhancement of the expression of histocompatibility antigens	
Mouse	Inhibition of antibody formation *in vitro*	
Mouse	Inhibition of sensitization to sheep erythocytes and the expression of delayed type hypersensitivity in mice	
Mouse	Enhancement of natural killer cell activity *in vivo* and *in vitro*	
Mouse	Enhancement of cell sensitivity to the toxicity of polyI: polyC	
Human fibroblast	Enhancement of spontaneous cytotoxicity of lymphocytes	Einhorn (1980)
Human leukocyte	Enhancement of natural "killer" lymphocytes	Berg and Heron (1980c)
Human leukocyte	Enhancement of mixed lymphocyte reaction	
Human leukocyte	Enhancement of HLA expression on lymphocytes	

[a] Nonantiviral activities other than inhibition of cell growth which is shown in Table III.

IV). A most important finding in the contribution by Gresser *et al.* (1979) is that pure mouse interferon inhibits the growth of a transplantable tumour in mice. It seems quite clear (finally) that the same protein that induces the antiviral activity causes a variety of biologic effects. The molecular mechanisms by which the interferons cause the various nonantiviral effects are unknown. The investigation of these mechanisms will undoubtedly be an area of very active research in the future as more pure interferons become available.

IV CONCLUSION

My main interest during my participation in interferon research has been purification and characterization which explains this somewhat prejudiced account. Currently, there is excellent research ongoing in these areas in a number of laboratories and the acquisition of knowledge should accelerate. There are now two conclusions about the interferons with which there can be no argument: (1) interferons can be obtained pure and the protein studied;

(2) interferons can cause multiple biologic effects that are apparently separate and distinct from the antiviral activity.

The characterization of the interferons is being retarded by only one problem; there is not enough of these scarce proteins. Clearly, progress would be much faster if milligrams of a pure interferon were available instead of micrograms. This may change, however, if production of an interferon by a micro-organism, via cloning, can be developed; and/or if production by better and larger animal cell cultures can be achieved. In any case, during the next years we should learn a great deal about the interferon proteins and their genes. We will be able to probe the antiviral mechanism and the other biologic effects with more confidence using pure interferons. There are many questions for which answers should be forthcoming. What are the sequence homologies among a number of interferons at the amino acid level? Does the homology have any meaning in terms of biological activity? How are the four (at least) human interferon genes arranged within a cell? Does the family of proteins we call the interferons have a broader role in cellular and multicellular regulation that we have not discovered? Are there more interferons in the same animal, (e.g. human) yet to be discovered? These questions are not original to me for they have been asked by many. Their answers may come much sooner than we previously thought possible.

Finally, has the time spent in the purification of an interferon with its accompanying travails and disappointments been worth it. The answer is yes, because of the intellectual rewards and because of the friends involved in a common quest. There has been good competition and almost everyone has had an unfailing good sense of humour. There is yet, however, a basic need in interferon research that has not been met. We need pure "mock-interferon". I have heard that several groups are attempting to obtain pure "mock-interferon" and that they will report their results in the near future. A friend tells me that he is cloning the gene for "mock-interferon". I am anxiously awaiting his results.

V REFERENCES

Berg, K. and Heron, I. (1980a). *Scand. J. Immunol.* **11**, 489–502.

Berg, K. and Heron, I. (1980b). *J. gen. Virol.* in press.

Berg, K. and Heron, I. (1980c). *Ann. N.Y. Acad, Sci.* in press.

Berthold, W., Tan C. and Tan, Y. H. (1978). *J. biol. Chem.* **253**, 5206–5212.

De Maeyer-Guignard, J., Tovey, M., Gresser, I. and De Maeyer, E. (1978). *Nature* **271**, 622–625.

Einhorn, S. (1980). *J. clin. lab. Immunol.* **3**, 35–38.

Evinger, M., Rubinstein, M. and Pestka, S. (1980). *Ann. N.Y. Acad, Sci.* in press.

Fantes, K. H. and Furminger, I. G. S. (1967). *Nature* **216**, 71–72.

Gresser, I., De Maeyer-Guignard, J., Tovey, M. and De Maeyer, E. (1979). *Proc. natn. Acad. Sci. U.S.A.* **76**, 5308–5312.

Hunkapiller, M. W. and Hood, L. E. (1978). *Biochemistry* **17**, 2124.
Hunkapiller, M. W. and Hood, L. E. (1980). *Science* **207**, 523–525.
Iwakura, Y. and Yonehara, S. and Kawade, Y. (1978). *J. biol. Chem.* **253**, 5074–5079.
Kawakita, M., Cabrer, B., Taira, H., Rebello, M., Slattery, E., Weideli, H. and Lengyel, P. (1978). *J. biol. Chem.* **253**, 598–602.
Knight, E., Jr (1975). *J. biol. Chem.* **250**, 4139–4144.
Knight, E., Jr (1976a). *Proc. natn. Acad. Sci. U.S.A.* **73**, 520–523.
Knight, E., Jr (1976b). *Nature* **262**, 302–303.
Knight, E., Jr. Hunkapiller, M. W., Korant, B. D., Hardy, R. W. F., and Hood, L. E. (1980). *Science* **207**, 525–526.
Mantei, N., Schwarzstein, M. M., Streuli, M., Panem, S., Nagata, S. and Weissmann, C. (1980). *Gene* in press.
Nagata, S., Taira, H., Hall, A., Johnsrud, L., Streuli, M., Ecsödi, J., Boll, W., Cantell, K. and Weissman, C. (1980). *Nature* in press.
Okamura, H., Berthold, W., Hunkapiller, M. W., Hood, L. E., Smith-Johannsen, H., Inoue, H. and Tan, Y. H. (1980). *Biochemistry* in press.
Paucker, K., Cantell, K. and Henle, W. (1962). *Virology* **17**, 324–334.
Rubinstein, M., Rubinstein, S., Familletti, P. C., Miller, R. S., Waldman, A. A. and Pestka, S. (1979). *Proc. natn. Acad. Sci. U.S.A.* **76**, 640–644.
Stewart II, W. E. (1979a). "The Interferon System." Springer, New York.
Stewart II, W. E. (1979*b*). *In* "Interferon 1979 Volume 1" (Ed. I. Gresser), pp. 29–52. Academic Press, London.
Taira, H., Broeze, R. J., Jayaram, B. M., Lengyel, P., Hunkapiller, M. W. and Hood, L. E. (1980). *Science* **207**, 528–530.
Tan, Y. H., Barakat, F., Berthold, W., Smith-Johannsen, H. and Tan, C. (1979). *J. Biol. Chem.* **254**.
Taniguchi, T., Ohno, S., Fujii-Kuriyama, Y. and Muramatsu, M. (1980a). *Gene* in press.
Taniguchi, T., Mantei, N., Schwarzstein, M., Nagata, S., Muramatsu, M. and Weissmann (1980b). *Gene* in press.
Zoon, K. C., Smith, M. E., Bridgen, P. J., ZurNedden, D. and Anfinsen, C. B. (1979). *Proc. natn. Acad. Sci. U.S.A.* **76**, 5601–5605.
Zoon, K. C., Smith, M. E., Bridgen, P. J., Anfinsen, C. B., Hunkapiller, M. W. and Hood, L. E. (1980). *Science* **207**, 527–528.

Effects of Interferons on Cell Growth and Function

JOYCE TAYLOR-PAPADIMITRIOU

Imperial Cancer Research Fund, Lincoln's Inn Fields, London, UK

I BACKGROUND AND INTRODUCTION

Although interferons were reported to inhibit cell multiplication as early as 1962 (Paucker *et al.*, 1962) it is only quite recently that this effect and effects on other cell functions have been accepted as real phenomena. There are probably two main explanations for the reluctance to accept growth inhibition by interferon as part of its action. Firstly, it had been discovered as an antiviral agent and most workers in the field would have liked to believe that its only effect was to inhibit viral multiplication and that in fact it had no effect on cells, thus making it an ideal agent to be used in the clinic. A second and more objective reason for not accepting growth inhibition by interferon as a real effect was that the preparations of interferon being used at the time were very impure. In fact they were preparations of other materials contaminated with small amounts of interferon, so that the objection that other factors could actually be affecting cell function was a reasonable one. Clearly purified preparations of interferons were required to decide whether the same molecule could in fact have effects on cells as well as inhibiting virus proliferation. Since such purified preparations of both mouse and human interferons have now been obtained and have been shown to have effects on cells (as well as effects on virus growth), I am in the novel position of being able to write about these effects of interferons on cell functions without having first to devote some time to persuading readers that the phenomena under discussion exist.

Before embarking on a discussion of the various effects of interferon on cell function, it is worth while to examine briefly how interferons began to wander from the straight road of simple antivirals to follow the many side-roads that are now mapped. Fairly soon after the discovery of interferons as antiviral agents, work on oncogenic viruses led to the discovery that interferon preparations could inhibit transformation and production of tumours by these viruses. Subsequent work with chemically induced and transplantable tumours, showed that interferons could also inhibit the growth of tumours which did not have an apparent viral aetiology (for review see Gresser and Tovey, 1978). Since it was known that interferon could inhibit cell multiplication, it was natural to assume that interferons were inhibiting the development of some tumours by directly inhibiting the proliferation of the tumour cells. The elegant demonstration coming from Ion Gresser's laboratory (Gresser *et al.*, 1972) that L_{1210} cells, which were resistant to interferon's anticellular effect *in vitro*, could be inhibited *in vivo*, showed that factors other than direct inhibition of cell growth must be operating to inhibit tumour growth *in vivo*. This observation led to the demonstration by Lindahl and Gresser and their colleagues that interferons have profound effects on the cells of the immune system (Lindahl *et al.*, 1972; Lindahl–Magnusson *et al.*, 1972) and can also affect the expression of surface antigens on target cells (Lindahl *et al.*, 1973). It is now clear from their work and from the work of other investigators, that interferon is able to regulate the function and division of the effector cells of the immune system and to affect the target cells by acting on their surfaces (for review see Gresser, 1977; Balkwill, 1979). From a combination of *in vivo* and *in vitro* studies, a picture has emerged which shows an enormous range of cell functions to be affected by interferons. These are listed in Table I and the phenomena which have

TABLE I Effects of Interferon on Cell Functions

Inhibition of	
1* Cell division in:	
L cells	Paucker *et al.* (1962)
stimulated lymphocytes	Lindahl Magnusson *et al.* (1972)
regenerating liver	Frayssinet *et al.* (1972)
bone marrow	van't Hull *et al.* (1978)
epithelial cells	Balkwill *et al.* (1978)
2* Tumourigenicity	Gresser *et al.* (1972) Gresser and Tovey (1978)
3* Antibody formation *in vivo* and *in vitro*	For reviews see Gresser (1977) Balkwill (1979)
4* Delayed hypersensitivity reaction	De Maeyer and De Maeyer-Guignard (1977)
5 Thymidine uptake in L_{1210} cells	Brouty-Boye and Tovey (1978)
6 Dimethyl sulphoxide induced differentiation in Friend cells	Rossi *et al.* (1977a, b)
7 Insulin induced differentiation of 3T3 cells to adipocytes	Grossberg and Keary (1980)
8 Steroid inducible glycerol-3-phosphate	Illinger *et al.* (1976)
9 Steroid inducible tyrosine aminotransferase in hepatoma cells	Beck *et al.* (1974)
10 Glutamine synthetase in chick neural retina	Matsuno and Shirasawa (1978)
11 Induction of ornithine decarboxylase activity in fibroblasts by serum growth factors and tumour promoters	Sreevalson *et al.* (1979) Sreevalson *et al.* (1980)
12 Serum induced release of plasminogen activator	Schroder *et al.* (1978)
13 Maturation of human monocytes to macrophages	Lee and Epstein (1980)
Enhancement of	
1 Phagocytosis by macrophages	Donahoe and Huang (1976)
2 Cytotoxicity of sensitized lymphocytes	Lindahl *et al.* (1972)
3 Activity of natural killer cells	Trinchieri and Santoli (1978)
4 Production of antibody	Gisler *et al.* (1974)
5 Expression of surface antigens	Lindahl *et al.* (1973)
6 Expression of carcino-embryonic antigen	Attallah *et al.* (1979)
7* Producing of interferon (priming)	Stewart *et al.* (1971)
8 Induction of aryl hydrocarbon hydroxylase	Nebert and Friedman (1973)
9 IgE-mediated histamine release by basophils	Ida *et al.* (1977)
10 Synthesis of t-RNA methylase	Rozee *et al.* (1969)
11 Synthesis of prostaglandins	Yaron *et al.* (1977)
12 Synthesis of ketosteroids in adrenal cells	Chany *et al.* (1980)
13* Cytotoxicity of dsRNA	Stewart *et al.* (1972)
14 Beat frequency of myocardial cells	Blalock and Stanton (1980)
15 Excitability of cultured neurones	Calvet and Gresser (1979)

been demonstrated with purified mouse interferon (Gresser *et al.*, 1979) have been marked with an asterisk. It seems probable that the other functions which have so far only been shown to be affected by crude or partially purified interferons, will soon be shown to be also affected by the purified molecule.

II INTERFERON AS A HORMONE

An examination of the functions which can be affected by interferon in Table I shows how far interferons have moved from being specific antivirals. Thus, while still defining the interferons by their ability to inhibit virus growth, it seems reasonable at this point to regard them as hormones, similar, in some respects to known polypeptide hormones or growth factors (e.g. insulin, epidermal growth factor, prolactin or vasopressin), but with important differences. This is not a new concept, having been put forward by several people in different ways (Chany, 1976; Gresser, 1977; Grollman *et al.*, 1978). Moving the interferons into a class of substances known to have pleiotypic effects on cells does not simplify the problem of how interferon can affect so many cell functions, but makes the question recognizable, as one that has been asked for many years about the mechanism of hormone action. The similarities between interferon and many other polypeptides with affect cell function are:

(1) They interact with specific receptors in the cell membrane, as the first step in affecting cell function.
(2) They may affect cell proliferation in a wide variety of cell types.
(3) They can affect a range of cell functions, depending on the cell type and its stage of differentiation.

Interferons differ from all the other polypeptide hormones or growth factors in being glycoproteins and in two important respects. Firstly, they inhibit the multiplication of a wide range of viruses, and secondly they inhibit (rather than stimulate) cell proliferation. This last property of the interferons make them the first well defined negative growth factors. There are many proteins and peptides which can stimulate cell proliferation in a wide variety of cells and some of these can also affect specific cell functions in certain cell types. For example the neurohypophyseal nonapeptide vasopressin, which can promote Na^+ transport in some tissues, can act as a potent mitogen in 3T3 cells (Rozengurt *et al.*, 1979). Insulin is another hormone which affects specific functions in some tissues, but with general growth promoting properties for cells in culture. However, no naturally occurring substances have been previously characterized as regulating cell growth by inhibiting it. The chalones, a group of nontoxic cell growth inhibitors, reputed to have tissue specificity, have been investigated for longer than the interferons but have remained largely undefined. It is probably fair to say that the biological assay for the antiviral activity for interferons has been invaluable in characterizing these molecules which also have important regulatory effects on cell growth and metabolism. There may be other naturally occurring negative growth factors which do not inhibit virus growth but with inhibition of cell growth as the only assay, their identification and characterization may be more difficult.

As regulators of the immune response, interferons can also be viewed as hormones. Interferons are produced in the course of various immune reactions, and can have a range of enhancing or inhibitory effects on the immune system *in vitro* and *in vivo* (see Table I). As a generalization, interferons appear to be able to inhibit sensitization and proliferation of effector cells, while enhancing many of their differentiated functions (for reviews see Gresser, 1977; Balkwill, 1979). A critical evaluation of these phenomena and their relation to effects of lymphokines however, demands an intimate acquaintance with the complexities of regulation of growth and function in haemopoietic cells. We will therefore refer to these effects of interferons only where they relate to the general discussion, not forgetting their importance both in basic studies on the immune system and in the antitumour effect of interferon.

III INTERACTIONS OF INTERFERONS WITH THE CELL MEMBRANE

Having said that interferons resemble polypeptide hormones in inducing their effects by first interacting with the cell membrane, one has to admit then that most of the evidence supporting this statement is not directly related to interferons effects on cell function. There is however fairly convincing data to show that: (1) interaction with receptors is necessary to its antiviral effect; (2) changes in the cell membrane can be detected after interferon interacts with it.

A Evidence for Interaction with Membrane Receptors

Perhaps the most convincing evidence that interferon must start its action from the outside of the cell is that anti-interferon serum blocks the ability of poly IC to protect cells against virus infection (Vengris *et al.*, 1975). Since 90% of the cells in this experiment were producing interferon, the interpretation that interaction with the outer cell membrane is a necessary step in interferon's antiviral action is almost certainly correct. What do we know about this interaction?

Inhibition of the antiviral effect by pre-incubation with gangliosides and by the addition of cholera toxin or thyroid stimulating hormone (Besançon and Ankel, 1974; Grollman *et al.*, 1978) have implicated gangliosides in the functioning of a membrane receptor for interferon. Moreover, the ability of added gangliosides, when incorporated into the membrane, to increase the sensitivity of cells to the antiviral effect of interferon, (Vengris *et al.*, 1976) is a direct demonstration that they play some role in membrane interferon interactions. Many polypeptide hormones interacting with cells at the membrane do so with a specific glycoprotein receptor however. Such, a protein has certainly not been directly characterized as the interferon receptor but its existence is inferred from studies on interferon binding in membrane vesicles (Grollman *et al.*, 1978). Thus Grollman *et al.* (1978) have shown that the inclusion of a protein extract (free of glycolipid) of KB cells into liposomes confers on them the ability to bind TSH and cholera toxin and the binding is inhibited by interferons. Since KB cells are insensitive to the action of interferon, and have a very low content of gangliosides in their membranes, these workers suggest that the functional receptor for interferon (and for certain hormones) is made up of glycoprotein and glycolipid.

Genetic studies (Chany *et al.*, 1973; Tan *et al.*, 1973; Chany *et al.*, 1975) and studies with interferon bound to Sepharose beads (Ankel *et al.*, 1973) implicate a membrane interaction of interferon with the cell, but do not give information which would necessarily characterize the nature of the membrane receptor, which could be glycoprotein, glycolipid or both. Tan originally allocated the gene (or genes) governing sensitivity to interferon action in human cells to chromosome 21 by showing that in mouse–human somatic hybrids, sensitivity to human interferon segregated with indophenol oxidase. There is now fairly strong evidence to support the idea that sensitivity to interferons antiviral effect is directed by chromosome 21, most of it coming from examining the sensitivity of cells trisomic for this chromosome to the antiviral action of interferon (Tan *et al.*, 1974; Chany *et al.*, 1975; De Clercq, 1978). Arguments supporting the idea that chromosome 21 codes (directly or indirectly) for a membrane receptor for interferon have been, to my mind subjective. However, two pieces of evidence suggest that this in fact may be the case. The first is the reported inhibition of interferon action by an antibody to a membrane component coded for by chromosome 21 (Revel *et al.*, 1976). The other important observation is that a mouse–human hybrid carrying only chromosome 21 is sensitive to human interferon, and moreover, the phosphorylated 67K protein now implicated in interferon's antiviral action, is of mouse origin (Slater *et al.*, 1978). Taken together these experiments strongly suggest that chromosome 21 codes for a membrane protein or a protein involved in the synthesis of a membrane component (e.g. glycolipid) which is necessary for a functional interaction of interferon with the membrane. The high level of interferon required for induction of the antiviral state in the hybrid cells make the interpretation of the data somewhat less clear, since human interferon can act on mouse cells and the sensitivity of the parent mouse line is not reported.

The interactions of interferon with the cell membrane which lead to growth inhibition or effects on cell functions are almost completely unexplored. Experiments with trisomic cells have led to the conclusion that chromosome 21 also codes for sensitivity to interferons' growth inhibitory effect (Tan, 1976) and to its effect on monocytes (Epstein *et al.*, 1980). However the priming, and the increased sensitivity to dsRNA induced by interferon are not increased in cells trisomic for chromosome 21 (De Clercq *et al.*, 1975). It is not immediately clear to me why the important observation on inhibition of the antiviral action by an antibody to a membrane component (coded for by chromosome 21) has not been pursued and extended to seeing whether other interferon-induced effects are inhibited by the same antibody.

B Changes in Membranes of Interferon-treated Cells

Table II lists the changes in cell membranes which have been reported to result from interferon-treatment. All in all, it would seem that interferon does induce changes in cell membranes; how specific these changes are remains to be seen. Some of them are late events (e.g. effects on budding

Table II Changes in Cell Membranes Induced by Interferons

Increased expression of surface antigens	Lindahl *et al.* (1973)
Increased net negative charge	Knight and Korant (1977)
Increase in intramembrane particles	Chang *et al.* (1978)
Increased binding of lectins	Huet *et al.* (1974)
Changes in ion transport in membrane vesicles	Grollman *et al.* (1978)
Changes in uptake of thymidine	Broute-Boye and Tovey (1978)
Inhibition of binding of cholera toxin and TSH	Kohn *et al.* (1976)
Inhibition of cap formation of surface components on lymphocytes	Matsuyama (1979)
Decreased exposure of oligosaccharide moities of some gangliosides	Grollman *et al.* (1978)
Stimulation of adenyl cyclase activity	Friedman and Pastan (1969)
Effects on release of mouse leukaemia virus particles infected cells	Billieau *et al.* (1973), Friedman and Ramseur (1974), Chang *et al.* (1977), Pitha *et al.* (1976)
Effects on incorporation of glycoprotein (G) and membrane protein (M) into Vesicular Stromatitis Virus	Maheshwari *et al.* (1980)

of viruses) and may be dependent on interferon-induced protein synthesis. Others however happen very quickly, are readily reversible upon removing interferon, and probably reflect a change in the membrane resulting from interaction of interferon with its receptor. The reported changes in ion fluxes induced by interferon across membrane vesicles, and in thymidine uptake in whole cells could be analogous to the changes induced in uptake of ions and small molecules by polypeptide growth factors and tumour promoters (Rozengurt, 1979). These occur within seconds after interaction of the growth factor with the cell membrane and are protein synthesis independent events. Although interferons can successfully inhibit the growth stimulatory effects of growth factors and tumour promoters however, we have found that the stimulation of early uptake of ions, nucleosides and sugars by these factors is not affected by interferon. The immediate effects on uptake of ions and small molecules therefore resulting from cell interaction with growth factors appear to be dominant over any interferon induced effects, even though the inhibitory effect of interferon on cell growth is evident. The results on uptake of ions in whole cells treated with interferon are not entirely in agreement with those obtained using vesicles, and perhaps some care should be exercised in translating effects obtained with vesicle preparations to whole cells.

Perhaps the most interesting phenomenon which is probably a result of an effect on the cell membrane is the effect of interferon on the assembly or release of murine leukaemia virus (MLV) virus particles. In the various cell lines and strains used in these studies, it has been shown that while interferon inhibits the production of infectious virus, intracellular events involved in virus replication, are not affected. In some cases interferon treated cells showed an increased number of membrane associated particles, suggesting budding was inhibited; in others particles were released but many were noninfectious. Similar observations have now been made on interferons effect on Vesicular Stomatitis Virus production; again many noninfectious particles with defective glycoprotein spikes are released from interferon treated cells. Thus, the reduction in infectious virus production in some of those viruses which use host cell membrane components in their assembly, may be attributable in part to a direct effect of interferon on the cell membrane—an unexpected twist.

C Potential Interest of Interferon–Membrane Interactions

The study of the interaction of interferon with the cell membrane, I believe is an area of great interest and importance. Now that purified interferons are available, it should be possible to investigate the interaction directly by following binding of labelled protein. (Using biologically active, purified ^{125}I-labelled mouse interferon, Aguet (1980) has shown that sensitivity to interferon may be related to specific binding of the protein.) Moreover, it may be feasible to raise monoclonal antibodies to membrane antigens involved in interferon binding and action. With these techniques, it should be possible to ask whether the same receptor positioned topographically in the same way is involved in initiating all of the interferon mediated effects. There are few if any naturally occurring molecules which exhibit quite the extensive range of actions reported for interferons. It will be very interesting to see whether the same membrane interaction can induce them all. Different parts of the molecule of human interferon appear to interact with receptors on cells of different species (Paucker *et al.*, 1975). This raises the possibility that different cell types, within the same species may present a different receptor to the interferon molecule, allowing them (the cells) to respond in a different way. Even the same receptor, positioned differently in the membranes of the various cell types could result in a variety of interactions which might perturb the membrane differently, and consequently affect various aspects of cell metabolism.

The interaction of polypeptide hormones and growth factors with membrane receptors, the internalization of the complex and the fate of the internalized hormone are areas of intensive investigation. In considering interferon actions within the framework of polypeptide hormones, many concepts and experimental approaches can be borrowed from this rapidly developing area. Thus it will be important to ask whether internalization of interferon and degradation of the internalized hormone are crucial to its actions on cell growth and function. The experiments showing that interferon bound to Sepharose beads can induce an antiviral state do not exclude the possibility that a small fraction of the interferon is split off from the beads upon association with the membrane. Again, radioactively labelled preparations of purified interferons will allow direct investigation of internalization and degradation of the molecule.

IV INHIBITION OF CELL PROLIFERATION

A General Features of Inhibition of Cell Growth *In Vitro*

It is still stated by some investigators that interferons inhibit the growth of tumour cells more than that of normal cells. While this may apply in some cases (Strander and Einhorn, 1977), it is not generally true. On the contrary, if 3T3 cells are compared to SV_{40}-transformed 3T3 cells, or normal human mammary epithelial cells to breast cancer cells, the normal cells are at least as sensitive to the growth inhibitory effect of interferon as their transformed or malignant counterparts (Balkwill *et al.*, 1978; Taylor-Papadimitriou, unpublished data). In fact the effect of interferons on cell proliferation appears to be as general as the antiviral effect, all cells of the relevant species being sensitive to some degree or other. It should be borne in mind however that very few cell lines have been looked at with pure interferons.

The relative effectiveness of the different human interferons, fibroblast, leukocyte and immune, as growth inhibitors, may differ. Most of the data available from *in vitro* studies have been obtained using Type I interferons and it would seem that the growth of most cells is inhibited by these interferons in concentrations around 100–1000 units/ml. Some cells, such as Daudi lymphoblastoid cells (Adams *et al.*, 1975) are affected by lower concentrations and some are unaffected by higher concentrations. Also, growth inhibition can be seen with much lower levels if interferon is cultured for long periods of time with the cells. Although the levels of interferons required for growth inhibition are generally higher than those required for the antiviral effect, they are in the nanogram range and thus comparable to, or less than, the levels of growth factors (e.g. epidermal growth factor (EGF), fibroblast growth factor (FGF)) required to stimulate cell growth *in vitro*. Thus, even as inhibitors of cell proliferation, the interferons show a high specific activity.

While interferons can be cytotoxic if applied in high concentrations for long periods of time to cells in very sparse culture, the inhibitory effect is usually reversible upon removal of the interferon (Gresser *et al.*, 1970; Balkwill *et al.*, 1978). It is this ability of interferons to regulate cell growth, i.e. their cytostatic, rather than cytotoxic effect which makes them so interesting in the study of growth regulation.

B Role of Inhibition of Cell Growth by Interferon in Host Defence Mechanisms

The natural stimuli which appear to be effective in stimulating the production of interferons in animals are foreign antigens, of which viruses form a specially effective group. Viruses can stimulate the production of Type I interferons in many cell types including lymphocytes. Although it is generally thought that these interferons are more effective in inhibiting viral replication than cell proliferation, the levels produced by lymphocytic choriomeningitis virus can be high enough to effect permanent damage to organs in the newborn mouse—presumably by affecting cell proliferation or cell function (Riviere *et al.*, 1977). It is therefore conceivable that in early virus infection, enough circulating or localized interferon may be produced to inhibit the growth of some cells. This would be useful in stopping the integration of an oncogenic virus, but it is hard to think of any other purpose it would serve in augmenting the hosts defence mechanism against virus infection.

Type II interferons produced by lymphocytes in response to an antigenic stimulus could, by inhibiting the growth of the cells carrying the antigens (viral or tumour) form part of the so called immune surveillance mechanism of the host. Is this likely? Perhaps in combination with their ability to increase recruitment of natural killer cells (Saksela *et al.*, 1979) and enhance the expression of surface antigens on tumour cells, interferons could play such a role. It is interesting that the interferon produced by sensitized lymphocytes in the mixed lymphocyte reaction or by mitogen stimulated lymphocytes is Type II interferon (Valle *et al.*, 1975) while natural killer cells (NK) challenged with cells carrying foreign antigens apparently produce Type I (Trinchieri *et al.*, 1978). One could argue that the Type II interferon is primarily important in down regulation of the stimulated lymphocytes, while the NK produced Type I interferon serves to recruit more NK cells, and inhibit virus growth, and that neither play a major role in inhibition of growth of tumour cells. On the other hand the recent observations that Type I and Type II interferons act by different mechanisms (Dianzani *et al.*, 1980; Bourgeade *et al.*, 1980) allows the possibility that they may act synergistically in inhibiting cell growth so that a combined attack might be very effective in inhibiting tumour cell growth. With better preparations of Type II interferons available, this idea may be tested. My own prejudice would be that interferons quite probably play a role in the suppression of spontaneously arising cancer cells but more by affecting the functions of the effector cells of the immune system than by direct inhibition of tumour cell growth. The regulation of the proliferation of stimulated lymphocytes by interferons is almost certainly important in modulation of the immune response and will be discussed in a later section.

C Role of Growth-inhibition in Antitumour Effect of Exogeneously administered Interferons

Since interferons can enhance: (1) the functions of the cells of the immune system; (2) the expression of surface antigens on tumour cells, it is conceivable that inhibition of tumour growth by exogenously administered interferon occurs only through these indirect mechanisms and not at all through a direct effect on proliferation of the tumour cells. The inhibition of the *in vivo* growth of IF-resistant L_{1210} cells certainly indicates that interferon effects on the host are important in tumour inhibition. Is there any data to suggest that direct inhibition of tumour cell proliferation can also be involved? To test this one would need to follow the effect of interferon on tumour growth in an immune-suppressed host. Little has been done to analyse the development of tumours in an immune-suppressed allogeneic host. I know of only one study by Gresser and Bourali-Maury (1973), who reported that treatment of mice with antilymphocyte serum or X-irradiation did not abrogate the inhibitory effect of interferon on transplantable tumours. We have followed the effect of human interferon on the development of xenografts of human breast cancers in the nude mouse, and found that tumour development can be markedly suppressed (see Fig. 1 and Balkwill *et al.*, 1980). Although this

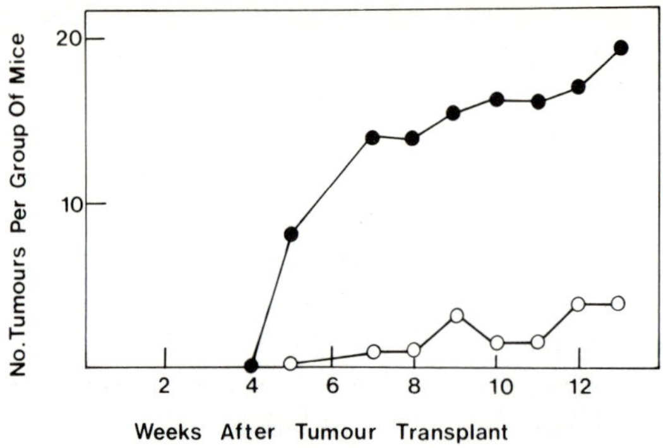

Fig. 1 Inhibition of development of human breast xenografts in nude mice. Human lymphoblastoid interferon (2×10^4 international units) (○——○) or phosphate buffered saline (●——●) was administered daily to each mouse (9 mice/group), which received 4 separate transplants of a human breast tumour at passage 2. The tumour originally developed 12 weeks after implantation from a biopsy specimen of a primary infiltrating carcinoma of the breast.

result cannot be directly translated to the situation of a tumour growing in an allogeneic host, it does suggest that a direct effect of interferon on cell proliferation can affect the development of a tumour mass. There is probably a great deal of information to be had from animal tumour model systems concerning the role of the various actions of interferon in tumour inhibition. These questions might be particularly relevant to problems related to the application of interferon in the clinic, since many patients who are candidates for interferon treatment might be in the category of being immune suppressed. This is a good reason for a continued commitment to work on the production of mouse interferons (both Type I and Type II) which are required in quite high levels for such *in vivo* experiments in mouse model systems.

D Inhibition of Normal Cell Growth *In Vivo*

If the effect of inhibition of cell proliferation is as general as it appears to be, we should ask two questions about its effect on normal cells *in vivo*. Firstly, how big a problem is inhibition of normal cell growth going to be in using interferon in the treatment of viral or malignant disease? Secondly, do interferons play a role in growth regulation in the normal functioning of the organisms?

1 Effects of exogeneously administered interferon. It is possible to give some answer to the first question by saying (as have other investigators) that the severity of the side-effects of interferon treatment have to be considered in relation to the severity of the disease and the condition and age of the patient.

Adverse effects resulting from inhibition of cell growth by interferon might be very serious in embryonic or neonatal development (Gresser *et al.*, 1975) or where extensive tissue regeneration is crucial to the patients survival (Frayssinet *et al.*, 1973). The major side-effect of leukocyte interferon, administered in clinical trials done so far, appears to be to depress the proliferation of cells in the bone marrow, and this effect is reversible, (Greenberg *et al.*, 1976). Compared to many of the chemotherapeutic agents in present use, some of which are carcinogenic as well as almost completely nonspecific in their cytotoxic effect, interferons may prove to be relatively benign. Until however, the effects of the long-term administration of interferon have been followed, it's use probably should be restricted to severe disease; even if it becomes available cheaply and in large amounts, administration for minor illnesses should perhaps be avoided.

2 Role of interferon in normal cell growth regulation. Whether interferons normally play any role in normal growth regulation *in vivo* is of course a very interesting question and it is possible to make some predictions based on the information available from *in vivo* and *in vitro* systems. While *in vitro* studies have shown a wide variety of cell types to be susceptible to the growth inhibitory effect of interferon, *in vivo* studies have focused predominantly on effects of interferon on cells of the immune system and on tumour cell growth. The available data showing inhibition of production of antibody forming cells, cytotoxic lymphocytes and bone marrow proliferation, strongly suggest that interferons are natural growth regulators in the immune response. The inhibition of the mitogenic stimulation of lymphocytes by the interferon produced by stimulated lymphocytes seems to be a fine example of a negative feedback, which would help to prevent the whole lymphocyte population becoming committed to producing grams of the same antibody or infinite numbers of cells sensitized to the same antigen. The reported sensitivity of myelomas (Mellstedt *et al.*, 1979) and lymphomas (Merigan *et al.*, 1978) to interferons's antitumour effect may be related to a natural role of interferons as growth regulators in these cells.

What about growth regulation by interferon of other cells in the body, those which make up organs, lining epithelia, stromal tissue? The cells which divide most frequently and at a steady rate in adult animals, are skin, and some lining epithelium. These are geared to divide at a certain rate and in healthy organisms this is equal to the rate of loss by shedding, by differentiation, or by other means. We have little information on the effect of interferon on those cell types and it would be useful to investigate interferon's effect on growth and differentiation of for example, human keratinocytes, which can now be grown in culture (Rheinwald and Green, 1975). Such studies might also yield information which would be relevant to any side-effects observed in the clinical use of interferon. Another type of growth which occurs in the adult animal is that which occurs under a specific stimulus, for a limited period of time and then stops. The growth of stimulated lymphocytes is an example of this kind of growth which is probably normally regulated at least in part by interferon. Other examples are the wounding response in skin, and the growth of the mammary gland at puberty and pregnancy. While topographical restraints are likely to be involved in the eventual inhibition of cell growth in these two examples, a role for interferons is not excluded. It is perhaps of interest that human mammary epithelial cells from the normal mammary gland are very sensitive to the growth inhibitory effect of leukocyte interferon. It has been suggested that interferons may show some tissue specificity in their action on cells (Einhorn and Strander, 1977) and this should be borne in mind when looking for a role for interferons in normal growth regulation.

If epithelial cells or fibroblasts were subject to growth control *in vivo* by interferon, perhaps one might expect them to produce it after mitogenic stimulation by serum or growth factors (by analogy with stimulated lymphocytes). We have not detected interferon produced by fibroblasts stimulated in this way but have no information as yet on epithelial cells. It would seem that the possibility of interferons being natural regulators of the growth of cells other than some of the haemopoietic stem cells, is not excluded, but there is no positive evidence to support this idea.

E Mechanisms involved in Interferon Induced Inhibition of Cell Proliferation

1 Possible approaches. Interferons were discovered in 1957 (Isaacs and Lindenmann, 1957) and it has taken the best part of two decades to make some real headway in unravelling the mechanisms involved in their antiviral action. The exciting discoveries of the last few years which implicate at least two induced enzymes in the antiviral action of interferon, were made possible largely because of the availability of the relatively simple cell free translation systems. I do not mean to imply that these are easy experimental systems to work with, merely that they effectively isolate a piece of the cell machinery, known to be important in the replication of all viruses, and thus allow the simplification necessary for the posing of questions which can be answered with less ambiguity than when asked in whole cells. The work in cell free systems could also be backed up by work with whole cells where virus replication could be isolated from cellular metabolism by the use of anti-metabolites, and thus anlaysed precisely and in depth. In short, the study of the inhibition of viral replication by interferon was helped by the fact that a great deal was learnt over the years about the replication of the different kinds of viruses and a specific stage of this replication could be studied in cell free systems.

The replication of mammalian cells is undoubtedly more complicated than the replication of the most complex viruses, and possible sites where interferons may act are multiple. How should one start to investigate what is in fact a very complex problem, made more diffuse by the lack of precise knowledge about the basic mechanisms involved in normal growth and growth control in various cell types. One approach is to start with the cell cycle, to try to break down the overall effect of interferons to specific phases of the cycle, and ultimately to effects on specific metabolic events within a phase. This is analogous to analysing the effects of interferon on virus replication by examining what it does to the various phases of the virus growth cycle (absorption, penetration, transcription, translation, assembly and release) with the difference that the phases of the cell cycle, particularly G_1 and G_2, which are gaps in information as well as in time, are ill defined in comparison with say translation of viral RNA. Despite these limitations, it is logical to look at the effect of interferons on the cell cycle, and already some studies have been done using various cell types. In our own work we have proceeded to try to analyse specific effects in G_1 in more depth by looking at molecular events.

Another approach is to focus on some particular aspect of cell metabolism or function which studies in other areas have suggested may be crucial in the control of growth, and look at interferon's effect on it. The advantage of this approach is that some important effects may be picked up quickly with the right combination of intuition and serendipity. The availability of *in vitro* culture systems for the study of cell proliferation of normal and virally transformed cells has meant that considerable progress has been made in characterizing factors affecting the growth of these cells (and produced by them). Serum can now be replaced by defined growth factors and hormones, and the molecular mechanisms involved in growth stimulation by such factors can be investigated. Also, differences in the behavioural properties of normal and transformed cells have been identified. Information coming from these investigations will undoubtedly be useful in helping to focus on specific aspects of cell metabolism in studying interferons anticellular effects.

Finally it is relevant to examine whether any of the molecular mechanisms now implicated in the antiviral effect of interferons are involved in the inhibition of cell growth.

2 Interferon and the cell cycle. An important feature of the cell cycle in proliferating eukaryotic cells is that the synthesis of DNA (S phase) occurs some time before the mitotic event (M). There may be a period (G_1) after M before the cell starts synthesizing DNA again, and quiescent cells are almost invariably found to be in G_1 (sometimes called G_0). Although G_1 is not an essential part of the cell cycle in rapidly proliferating cells, and cell mutants are available which have no G_1, this is the part of the cell cycle widely studied in those model systems where a mitogenic stimulus moves quiescent cells through G_1 to S. It may be more realistic to take the transition probability model of the cell cycle as being made up of phases of determinate or indeterminate length, (Smith and Martin, 1973) but for our purposes in discussing the relevant interferon data, the classical G_1, S, G_2, M, definition will suffice.

It is sensible to ask, whether interferon inhibits events in only one part of the cell cycle, since a block in a specific phase would immediately reduce the possibilities. This has been looked at with both asynchronously dividing cells (Killander *et al.*, 1976; Matarese and Rossi, 1977; Balkwill *et al.*, 1978) and with synchronized populations (Sokawa *et al.*, 1977; Balkwill *et al.*, 1978). The data available support the idea that interferon does not block the cells in one phase of the cell cycle but rather results in an extension of G_1 and $S + G_2$. The increased length in the cell cycle time (Collyn-d'Hooghe *et al.*, 1977) is therefore due to an extension of these phases. In fact S is usually affected less than G_1 and G_2 (Balkwill *et al.*, 1978) and the relative extent to which G_1 and G_2 are affected depends on the cell type (Balkwill and Taylor–Papadimitriou, 1978; Fig. 2).

The advantages of using quiescent cells, stimulated to divide synchronously by mitogens for analysing the metabolic events involved in the progression of the cell through the division cycle, are fairly obvious. After addition of mitogens, the whole cell population moves through G_1, and begins to synthesize DNA; the pre-replicative events, leading up to and necessary for DNA synthesis are occurring in all the cells at roughly the same time, and can therefore by analysed. The two systems which have been used widely to investigate pre-replicative events in this way have been quiescent fibroblast lines, stimulated usually by serum or polypeptide hormones (for reviews see Pardee *et al.*, 1978; Rozengurt, 1979) and lymphocytes stimulated by plant lectins (for review see Greaves and Janossy, 1972). The events which follow mitogenic stimulation and precede DNA synthesis can be classified as *early events* which happen within minutes after stimulation and do not depend on cellular protein synthesis, and *late events* which happen hours after stimulation by the mitogens and are protein synthesis dependent. The early events probably reflect the direct response of the cell membrane to interaction with the mitogen, and include increased transport of small molecules (ions, nucleotides, sugars) and changes in the intracellular level of cyclic AMP. The later events which depend on protein synthesis may also include secondary increases in uptake of ions and sugars, and in the activity of certain enzymes. Of these, ornithine decarboxylase is of particular interest since increases in the activity of this enzyme are invariably associated with the proliferative response of cells in culture, in regenerating tissue, in tumours, and also in tumour promotion (Janne *et al.*, 1978). Ornithine decarboxylase catalyzes the first rate limiting step in the synthesis of the polyamines, which

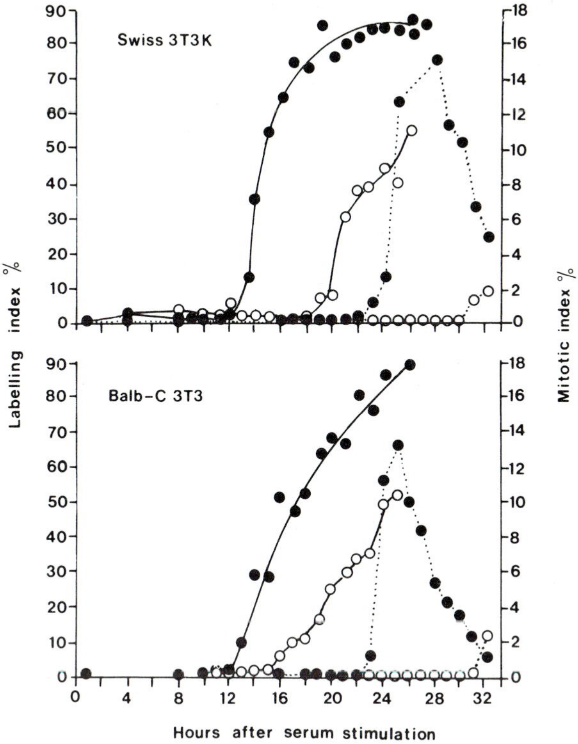

Fig. 2 Effect of interferon on entry into S phase and mitosis of serum stimulated synchronized Swiss 3T3K cells (top) and BALB/c 3T3 cells (bottom). Cells synchronized in G_1 by serum deprivation and growth to confluence were stimulated with fresh medium and 10% serum in the presence and absence of interferon (1000 U/ml). Labelling index in control cells (●——●) and in cells treated with interferon (○——○); mitotic index in control cells (●----●) and in cells treated with interferon ○----○. Reprinted by permission from *Nature* **274**, 798–800. Copyright © 1978 Macmillan Journals Limited.

are involved in the regulation of numerous cellular reactions, including translation and transcription (Janne, 1978).

When quiescent Swiss 3T3 cells are stimulated to grow with serum, the lag to S, which represents G_1 is extended by several hours, if interferon is added with the serum; G_2 is also lengthened by approximately 1–2 h, but the main effect is on G_1 (Fig. 2*a*). This provides a useful system therefore for the analysis of events in G_1 which are affected by interferon which are crucial to the initiation of DNA synthesis. A similar effect of interferon is obtained when insulin is used to stimulate growth in combination with vasopressin and epidermal growth factor, or with a tumour promoter (Sreevalson *et al.*, 1980). Results using 3T3 cells stimulated by mitogens are very clear; interferon appears to have no effect on the early increase in transport of ions, nucleosides or sugars, and selectively inhibits the increase in activity

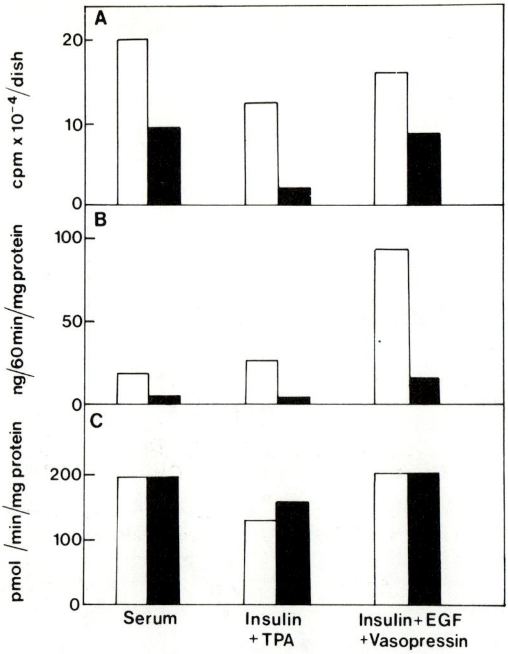

Fig. 3 Selective inhibition by interferon of ornithine decarboxylase activity in Swiss 3T3K cells stimulated from quiescence to growth by serum, or insulin (1·0 μg/ml) together with a tumour promoter tetradecanoylphorbol acetate (TPA) (100 ng/ml) or with epidermal growth factor (EGF 2·5 ng/ml) and vasopressin (10 ng/ml). (A) DNA synthesis measured at 48 h by ^{3}H-methyl thymidine incorporation. (B) Ornithine decarboxylase activity measured at 6 h (C) 2-Deoxyglucose uptake measured at 6 h. □, stimulated control cells; ■, interferon treated stimulated cells.

of ornithine decarboxylase. This is true whether the mitogens are serum, a combination of growth factors of a tumour promoter (Sreevalson *et al.*, 1979; 1980). The second phase of increase in glucose uptake, which is also protein synthesis dependent, is not inhibited by interferon (see Fig. 3), nor is the overall rate of protein synthesis (Sreevalson, unpublished data).

The fact that stimulation of DNA synthesis is inhibited by interferon whatever the mitogen indicates that a common interferon sensitive step is involved in stimulation of DNA synthesis by serum, hormones and tumour promoters. Interferon antagonism to mitogens is not limited to 3T3 cells. We have found that stimulation of DNA synthesis by mitogens as different as epidermal growth factor, oestrogen and cholera toxin (Stoker *et al.*, 1976; Taylor–Papadimintriou and Fentiman, 1980; Taylor–Papadimitriou *et al.*, 1980) is inhibited by interferon in human mammary epithelial cells (Fig. 4). It is therefore possible that interferons are inhibiting the same step (or steps) in a variety of cells stimulated by a wide range of mitogens. Identification of such a step (steps) might give us important information, not only about

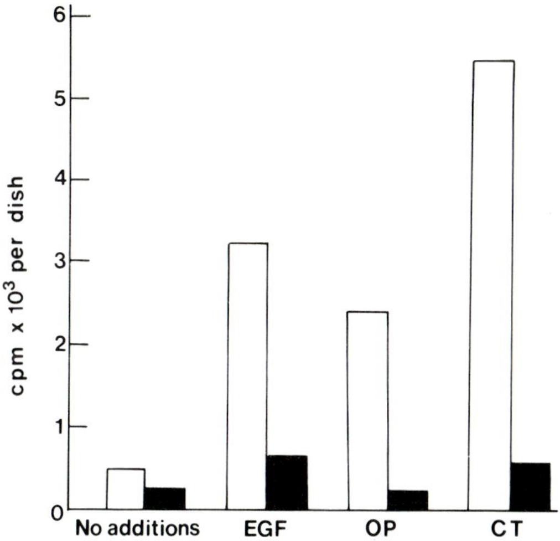

Fig. 4 Inhibition of DNA synthesis by interferon in human mammary epithelial cells stimulated by growth factors. Mammary epithelial cells from human milk were grown up with X-irradiated 3T6 feeders (Taylor-Papadimitriou *et al.*, 1980) and DNA synthesis estimated in the absence of serum and in the presence of growth factors by incorporation of ^{3}H-methyl thymidine into TCA in = soluble material. □, + growth factors; ■, growth factor + interferon (1000 U/ml).

interferon action but also about the mechanisms of growth promotion by mitogens. Since ornithine decarboxylase induction is always inhibited, one might think that this could be the interferon sensitive step crucial to DNA synthesis. An argument against this is that inhibition of ODC synthesis in human embryo skin fibroblasts does not result in inhibition of DNA synthesis in cells stimulated from quiescence by serum; the cells contain enough polyamines to get them through one cycle and are blocked in G_1 of the next (Hollta *et al.*, 1979). Whether this is a general phenomenon found in other cell types is not known. Even if induction of ODC is not the interferon sensitive step which is crucial to DNA synthesis, it is certainly important in cell proliferation and the inhibition of ODC induction is likely to play some role in the sustained inhibition of cell growth seen in interferon treated cells. Also, since the inhibition of ODC induction is selective, the system could be used to investigate the mechanism underlying the selectivity.

3 Effects on cell parameters changed in transformation and/or malignancy. Cell functions which change in malignancy may be related to the altered growth potential of malignant cells. It would be interesting, for pragmatic as well as academic reasons, to know whether interferon specifically affects any of the cell functions or parameters which change in malignancy. The problem here is knowing which parameters do actually change in malignant transformation. Work in fibroblast model systems have shown that virally transformed cells show: (1) an altered pattern of growth *in vitro* (review Hynes, 1979); (2) alterations in the cytoskeleton (Pollack *et al.*, 1975a); (3) altered secretion of proteins (Senger *et al.*, 1979) growth factors (Todaro and De Larco, 1978) and proteases (Pollack *et al.*, 1975b); (4) changes in membrane and surface components, particularly fibronectin (Hynes, 1976; Nicholson, 1976). Attempts to correlate changes in some of these parameters with tumourigenicity have shown that the formation of large colonies in agar, (Macpherson and Montagnier, 1964), i.e. anchorage independent growth, correlates best with tumourigenicity (Kahn and Shin, 1979; Steinberg and Pollack, 1979). Other parameters, such as production and retention of fibronectin, and increased production of plasminogen activity show incomplete correlation, and certain parameters describing growth such as loss of density dependent inhibition of growth, or requirement for mitogens, are probably hardly related at all to tumourigenicity. Even though this rather inconclusive information has been obtained mainly from fibroblast model systems, and may not be relevant to human epithelial cells, it still might be worth while to examine the effect of interferon on the whole list of parameters suggested by viral transformation systems as being important in growth control. It is a way of focusing the attempt to analyse the mechanism of interferon's growth inhibitory effect and could yield results which would direct us elsewhere. In this context the inhibition by interferon of release of plasminogen activator is of interest (Schroder *et al.*, 1978). The clonal growth of cells in agar, is in some instances very sensitive to interferons inhibitory effect (Gresser *et al.*, 1971), but to my knowledge no studies have been done comparing the dose of interferon required to inhibit growth of tumour or transformed cells on plastic and in agar. There may be a reproducibly stronger inhibition of anchorage independent growth of tumour cells—it would be easy to find out.

Chany and his colleagues have begun to examine the relationship between interferon and the cytoskeleton. So far, these studies have been mainly restricted to indirect experiments following the effects of agents which affect the cytoskeleton on the antiviral action of interferon. Agents like colchicine or vinblastin which disrupt the cytoskeleton inhibit the action of interferon. Sodium butryate, which is reported to promote organization of the cytoskeleton, enhances the action of interferon, particularly in transformed cells (Bourgeade and Chany, 1976; Bourgeade *et al.*, 1980). These experiments are very interesting and will no doubt be extended. Their clear interpretation presents some problems however since it depends on knowing: (1) exactly how the agents affecting interferon action act on the cytoskeleton (and if this is their only action); (2) what role the cytoskeleton plays in growth control and in the transmission of messages from membrane to cytoplasm.

The cytoskeleton is composed of those "semi-rigid and contractile elements which give structure to the cytoplasm and link the surface to the cytoskeleton"

(Allfreid and Potter, 1978). It is made up of microtubules, microfilaments (actin and myosin) and the trabecular network or cytoplasmic matrix. While there are certainly changes in the organization of microtubules and microfilaments observed in virally transformed fibroblasts (Pollock *et al.*, 1975*a*) the nature of the changes has yet to be clarified. Absolute levels of tubulin for example are not altered but assembly of the protein is (Rubin and Warren, 1979; Eichhorn and Peterkofsky, 1979). Furthermore it is not clear whether changes in cytoskeleton organization are a primary effect of transformation and whether they directly affect growth properties such as the capacity for anchorage-independent growth (O'Neil *et al.*, 1979; Folkman and Moscona, 1978). Surface components which interact with the cytoskeleton, such as fibronectin, (Perkins *et al.*, 1979) are also changed by transformation and it is possible that these changes are the primary ones which affect cytoskeletal organization. A complete study of how interferons affect the cytoskeleton, and through this cell growth and function, will involve examining its effects on each of the cytoskeletal elements and on their points of attachment at the surface and in the cytoplasm. A start has been made in this direction by some investigators (Chany *et al.*, 1980; Tamm *et al.*, 1980). However it is important to keep in mind that interpretation of results beyond the structural to the functional level will depend on progress in investigations following the role of the various components of the cytoskeleton in cell function.

In relation to its antigrowth effect it would be informative to look at the effect of interferons on the changes induced in the cytoskeleton by mitogens. The microtubules affect the transmission of the mitogenic signal induced by polypeptide growth factors, since the disruption of the microtubules in G_1 by colchicine enhances the stimulation of DNA synthesis by these factors (Friedkin *et al.*, 1979). Since colchicine inhibits the antiviral effect of interferon, it will be interesting to see whether the inhibition by interferon of the mitogenic effect of EGF is abolished by colchicine.

4 Interferon action and cyclic AMP. Some time ago Friedman and Pastan (1969) observed that interferons antiviral action is potentiated by dibutyryl cyclic AMP, and later it was reported that cyclic AMP levels are increased in interferon treated cells (Weber and Stewart, 1975; Meldolesi *et al.*, 1977). Cyclic AMP has been defined as a second messenger in the action of some hormones, which interact with the cell membrane (Sutherland, 1972) and for some year it was thought that increased levels of cyclic AMP were associated with reduced growth rates in some fibroblast systems (Rozengurt, 1979). The idea therefore that interferons action in inhibiting cell growth and affecting cell functions was mediated by an effect on membrane adenyl cyclase was an attractive one. More recent data however on cyclic AMP levels in interferon-treated cells, and on the role of cyclic AMP in growth regulation indicate that this possibility is unlikely. Tovey *et al.* (1980) find that cyclic AMP levels are not consistently altered until 24 h after addition of interferon when effects on cell multiplication are already apparent. Moreover, it is becoming obvious that the relation between growth rate and intracellular levels of cyclic AMP is not simple. The growth of some cell types, including Schwann cells, (Raffe *et al.*, 1978) human keratinocytes (Green, 1978) and human mammary epithelial cells (Taylor-Papadimitriou *et al.*, 1980) is markedly stimulated by cholera toxin or cyclic AMP analogues. In inhibiting the growth of these cell types interferon is hardly likely to be acting merely by raising levels of intracellular cyclic AMP. The observation that cyclic GMP levels are increased after interferon treatment (Tovey *et al.*, 1980) might be very interesting in view of the data showing reduced levels of cyclic GMP in proliferating cells (Miller *et al.*, 1975).

5 Relevance of molecular mechanisms involved in interferons antiviral effect. In the last five years, several laboratories have been successful in identifying specific proteins, induced in interferon treated cells, which almost certainly are involved in interferons antiviral effect (for review see Baglioni, 1979). Of these, the oligoadenylate synthetase (Kerr and Brown, 1978) which synthesizes a series of oligonucleotides with 2′-5′ phosphodiesterbonds, and the phosphokinase (Lebleu *et al.*, 1976; Roberts *et al.*, 1978; Zilberstein *et al.*, 1976) which phosphorylates the initiation factor eIF-2 (Farrell *et al.*, 1977) have been most studied. Both are activated by dsRNA and affect translation of viral messages, the synthetase by producing ppp $(2'\text{-p5A})_3$ which in turn activates a nuclease, and the kinase, by inactivation of eIF-2 by phosphorylation. An obvious development of this work is to ask if these systems are also involved in the growth inhibitory effects of interferon. Since both systems are activated by dsRNA, one would expect them to be amplified (as they appear to be) in virally infected cells. The question is do these mechanisms operate in uninfected interferon-treated cells to the extent that they could affect macromolecular synthesis and cell growth.

The role of the synthetase in interferon's effect on cell growth and in growth control in general has been investigated more than the kinase. This is probably partly because the effects of the product [2′-5′A] can be tested directly on cells (provided the cells are permeabilized). There is however one report by Wood and Hovanessian (1979) which attempts to relate kinase to interferons growth inhibitory effect. These investigators found that mouse embryonal carcinoma stem cells which are insensitive to interferons inhibitory effect on cell or virus growth do not produce the kinase after interferon treatment while the corresponding differentiated cells (whose growth is inhibited by interferon) do. This result merely allows the possibility of a role for the kinase in interferons growth inhibitory effect. There are undoubtedly many differences in the metabolic profile of the undifferentiated and the differentiated embryonal carcinoma cells, and any one could be related to acquired sensitivity to interferon.

It has been clearly shown that 2′-5′A does affect protein synthesis, and activates nuclease activity in intact cells (Williams and Kerr, 1978; Hovanessian *et al.*, 1979) thus excluding the possibility that the system is an artefact of the *in vitro* translation system where it was first observed. Moreover the dephosphorylated trimer (which can presumably pass through the cell membrane) has been shown to inhibit growth in Daudi cells (a lymphoblastoid line; Reisinger and Martin, 1980) and DNA synthesis in lectin stimulated lymphocytes (Kimchi *et al.*, 1979). The story which appears to be emerging from the lymphocyte work is very interesting and confirms the idea that interferon may be a natural growth regulator in these cells. Thus, Shimizu and Sokawa (1979) have found that normal lymphocytes contain high levels of 2′-5′ oligoadenylate synthetase, comparable to those found in interferon treated L cells. Con A stimulated lymphocytes which will go on to synthesize DNA and divide, apparently contain an inhibitor of the synthetase and interferon-treated cells contain higher levels of the enzyme (Kimchi *et al.*, 1979). The data accommodate the theory that 2′-5′A is normally involved in keeping lymphocytes quiescent, and is reduced after mitogenic stimulation. It is therefore quite likely that interferon inhibition of lectin induced DNA synthesis in lymphocytes could act through the 2′-5′A system.

These results should be considered in the light of other experiments following interferons effects on activation and proliferation of lymphocytes which suggest that it is sensitization rather than proliferation which is affected (for review see Gresser, 1977; Atallah *et al.*, 1979). There is now some evidence to indicate that the activation of T lymphocytes is a two step process consisting of: (1) exposure on the cell surface of functioning receptors for growth factors; (2) generation by accessory cells of growth factors which can interact with these surface receptors to induce cell proliferation and differentiation (Andersson *et al.*, 1979; Coutinho *et al.*, 1979). A ligand such as Con A, which is mitogenic for T cells can induce both the receptors on the T cells and the production of growth factors by other cells in the culture. Con A cannot however induce growth of the purified T cell blasts, which do not produced the growth factor. The studies following the effects of interferons on mitogenesis in lymphocytes would be consistent with the idea that the induction of the surface receptor and/or the growth factor is inhibited by interferon but the proliferation of blasts induced by the growth factor is not. It would be of interest to analyse in more detail the effect of interferons (and the role of 2′-5′A) on the various steps which appear to be involved in lymphocyte mitogenesis and proliferation, using conditions of growth which minimize cell death (Bernheim *et al.*, 1978).

Attempts to detect effects of 2′-5′A on the mitogenic effect of serum and growth factors in Swiss 3T3 cells, have met with little success (Taylor–

Papadimitriou and Kerr, unpublished data). The lack of inhibition could mean that the dephosphorylated oligonucleotide did not enter the cells, or it was not phosphorylated in the cells. An alternative explanation however is that fibroblasts do not normally use the 2′-5′A system in growth regulation and interferon inhibition of cell growth operates through some other mechanism in these cells.

6 Comments and conclusions. The observations with lymphocytes at different stages of proliferation and with fibroblasts, although fairly preliminary, emphasize the need to keep in mind the possible differences in growth regulation used by the various cell types. Multicellular organisms which develop from a single cell, through an embryonic stage to an independent organism, which grows and matures to become an adult, require cells to grow at different rates in response to different stimuli for different reasons and for varying numbers of cell divisions. While there undoubtedly will be features common to the mechanisms used in growth regulation by the various cells, there must also be important differences. One can again draw an analogy with virus replication. All the viruses use the machinery of the host cell to replicate their components, and growth cycles have common features; there are differences however depending on the virus type. Moreover, interferons appear to have pleiotypic effects, and affect several steps in viral replication some of which are important only to some viruses (e.g. budding of MLV).

It may turn out that interferons will tell us a great deal about growth regulation, by helping us to identify steps which are crucial to cell proliferation. A wide variety of cell types should be analysed, if possible at different stages of differentiation. In particular, it is quite important to look at epithelial cells, using the approaches discussed above since it is this cell type which gives rise to carcinomas, the major tumours in man.

V EFFECTS OF INTERFERON ON OTHER CELL FUNCTIONS

A look at Table I will show that apart from their effects on cell division, the interferons have been shown to affect a wide variety of cell functions, and that these functions may be inhibited in some cases, and in others enhanced, depending on the cell type. The regulation by interferons of the activities of the cells of the immune system are undoubtedly of enormous importance in the normal functioning of the host defense mechanism. Many of the interferon-related phenomena which have been reported have been observed *in vivo* or in mixed lymphocyte or leukocyte cultures. It will be important to work with homogeneous cell populations or at least defined populations if the role of interferons as a regulator in the immune response is to be investigated beyond the phenomenological level.

While the effect of interferons on other (non-haemopoietic) cell types, in culture may not reflect an *in vivo* role of the same importance as that of an immune regulator, these effects can be more easily studied at the cellular and molecular level, because of the experimental systems used. Let us consider these effects, under the headings of inhibitory or enhancing effects (Gresser, 1977).

A Inhibition of Cell Functions

Apart from its effect on cell division, interferons inhibitory effects on cell functions can mainly be classified as effects on the synthesis of induced enzymes or proteins (Table I). Differentiation in Friend cells means increased production of haemoglobin, and in adipocytes increased synthesis of enzymes involved in lipogenesis. The steroids induce a range of enzyme activities in different cell types, and ODC can also be considered an inducible enzyme, whose activity is increased by mitogens and tumour promoters. Even inhibition of lymphocyte mitogenesis by interferons may be due to inhibition of specific protein synthesis (growth factors or their receptors). In each of these cases, general protein synthesis is not affected, but the protein or enzyme under study is selectively inhibited by interferon. It is likely that the same molecular mechanisms are involved in the inhibition of the induction of specific proteins and in the inhibition of cell growth. This view assumes that the synthesis of proteins (other than ODC) induced by growth factors (polypeptides and steroids) and crucial to cell growth is also selectively inhibited by interferon. The idea of selective inhibition by interferon of the synthesis of specific inducible proteins, has the attraction of classifying most of the inhibitory effects as one phenomenon and leads to the conclusion that there is a common interferon-sensitive step in the regulation of synthesis of many inducible proteins in a wide range of cell types. We can now put a question which can be investigated experimentally namely, how does the selective inhibition operate?

As with interferon's antiviral action, an attempt has been made to distinguish between inhibition of the production of mRNA and inhibition of translation of the message. In the case of glutamine synthetase induction by steroids and DMSO-induced haemoglobin synthesis in Friend cells, an effect on the production of the respective message has been reported although an effect on translation of haemoglobin mRNA is also observed (Shirasawa and Matsuno, 1978; Rossi *et al.*, 1977a). In these studies, messenger RNA was measured directly, by translation in the first instance, and by hybridization with cDNA in the second. In our own work with ODC, indirect experiments with antimetabolites again suggest a major effect on transcription, although some effect on translation is also indicated (Sreevalson *et al.*, 1980).

Yau *et al.* (1978) have suggested that translation of viral mRNA's are selectively inhibited by interferon, because they initiate faster than cellular mRNAs and interferon inhibits elongation, which for these messages is rate limiting; the initiation rate for mRNAs whose translation is not readily inhibited by interferons is assumed to be rate limiting. To support these ideas Yau *et al.* report that cycloheximide (an inhibitor of elongation) selectively inhibits those viral mRNAs selectively inhibited by interferon, while pactomycin (an inhibitor of initiation of translation) inhibits host mRNA more than viral. Our own data following the effect of cyclohexamide and pactomycin on the induction of ODC by mitogens indicate that a similar mechan-

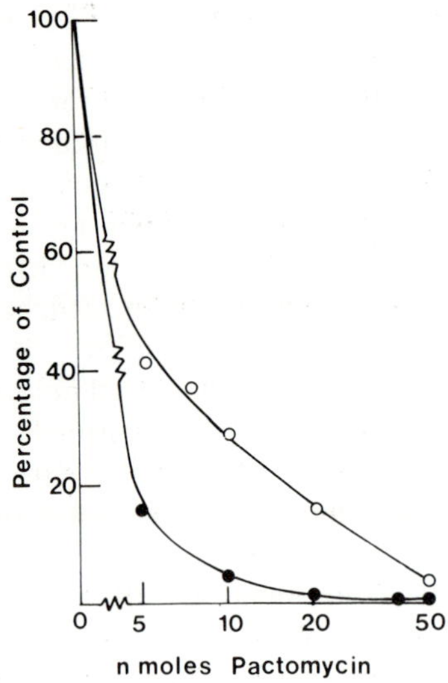

Fig. 5 Selective inhibition by pactomycin of ornithine decarboxylase activity induced by growth factors. Quiescent cells were stimulated with EGF, vasopressin and insulin (see Fig. 3) in the presence of various concentrations of pactomycin. Ornithine decarboxylase activity (●——●) and uptake of deoxyglucose (○——○) were measured 6 h later. The data are expressed as percentage of the values in the absence of pactomycin. The values for deoxyglucose uptake refer only to the proteinsynthesis dependent second phase.

ism is not operating in the selective inhibition of the synthesis of certain host proteins. Thus pactomycin inhibits the induction of ODC at concentrations which do not inhibit the protein synthesis-dependent increase in glucose transport (which also occurs after mitogenic stimulation and is not affected by interferon). The dose response curve for inhibition of the two activities is quite different (Fig. 5); cycloheximide shows no such selective inhibitory effect (Sreevalson *et al.*, 1979). It is possible that part of the selective inhibition of synthesis of host proteins by interferon could be attributed to a nonspecific inhibition of initiation of translation via the interferon induced kinase, which results in the inhibition of translation of some messages but not others. Clearly there are other explanations for the similar selectivity shown by pactomycin and interferon on ODC induction, and effects on translation cannot provide a complete explanation since transcription of messages is definitely inhibited.

B Enhancement of Cellular Functions

The cellular functions enhanced by interferon form a much more heterogeneous group than those which are inhibited. The increased sensitivity to double stranded RNA can probably be considered separate from the others, and explained in the light of the interferon induced enzymes, which inhibit translation of message and are activated by dsRNA. Perhaps the most coherent way to view the stimulatory effects of interferons on other functions, such as specific protein synthesis, release of histamine by basophils, synthesis of keto-steroids by adrenal cells, and (!) beat frequency of myocardial cells, is to consider them as wide ranging hormones, able to stimulate specific cell types to perform their specialized function. The variety of response is likely to be due to the different profile of metabolic reactions in the various differentiated cell types.

In order to study the molecular mechanism of this type of response, it will be easier to choose a system where the function enhanced is simple and defined like synthesis of a specific protein rather than complex and ill-defined (like phagocytosis, or cytotoxicity). In fact, interferons stimulation of their own synthesis might represent a good model system since interferon mRNA levels can be measured as well as interferon protein levels. There are certain obvious questions which spring to mind such as what is the role of 2′-5′A—can it reproduce the stimulatory effects of interferon as well as the inhibitory effects? Is the membrane receptor the same in the cell types giving the different responses? How effective are the different kinds of interferon on these various parameters. Most of the work has been done to date with Type I interferons. Now that immune interferons are becoming available in larger quantities, it will be possible to test their effects on all the cell functions known to be enhanced by Type I interferons. Finally it would be interesting to know whether interferon's action in affecting cell functions depends on synthesis of host messenger RNA in the same way as its antiviral action does (Taylor, 1964), although it is difficult to design an experiment to answer this question.

C Relevance to *In Vivo* Effects

While inhibition of proliferation of bone marrow cells has been emphasized as a major side effect of exogeneously administered interferon, it should be remembered that other undesirable responses have been observed in patients given high doses of interferons, and these could be related to some of the effects on cellular function just discussed. For example, the increase in heart beat sometimes observed may be due to a direct effect of interferon. Rigor, low blood pressure, pyrexia and general malaise and nausea are also quite common when high levels of interferon are administered repeatedly. In fact, there is a strong possibility that the symptoms experienced during viral infections may be caused by interferons rather than viruses themselves. Unless pure preparations of interferons are used clinically it is hard to interpret patient responses unequivocally, but it should be borne in mind that their various effects on cell functions could contribute to undesirable as well as desirable responses.

VI HOW MANY INTERFERONS?

The three human interferons commonly studied to date are leukocyte, fibroblast and immune (or Type II). It appears that the same cell type can produce more than one kind of interferon, and which is produced may depend on the inducing agent. Clearly it is going to be very important to sort out which cell types and which cell functions are affected and to what extent, by the different interferons. The suggestion that immune interferons are more potent growth inhibitors than Type I interferons is interesting. However, as comparisons are made on the basis of antiviral effects, and not on a per-mg-of-protein basis, the results obtained so far may merely indicate that immune interferons are relatively poor antiviral agents. There may be other molecules with growth inhibitory properties, but even less ability to inhibit viral replication. These will be difficult to identify because of the lack of a well defined assay, and begin to lose their definition as interferons. Even so there may be several genuine interferons produced by the effector cells of the immune system, and these must be interesting.

It is at first sight surprising that epithelial cells, which after all are the main target cell for common virus infections and spontaneous malignant transformation in man, have received so little attention by interferonologists. Some work has been done with interferon produced by human amnion (Fournier *et al.*, 1967; Chany *et al.*, 1973), but I am not aware of any studies on the characterization of this interferon. The justification for ignoring epithelial cells has been that they have been difficult to grow in culture and therefore to work with in a defined experimental situation. While they are still not as easy to grow as fibroblasts (or whatever the fast growing cell strains and lines in culture are) a variety of epithelial cells—even of human origin—can now be grown relatively easily in culture. I am referring to strains of cells which are close enough to their *in vivo* counterparts to retain their epithelial characteristics. Lines derived originally from epithelial cells after growth in culture for several years, and transferred as single cells, undoubtedly lose many properties associated with epithelial cells *in vivo* and should not be assumed to have retained any unless specifically demonstrated. However it is now possible to grow fairly large numbers of human keratinocytes, mammary epithelium, prostrate and bladder, and we should certainly begin to examine interferon production and action in early passage cultures of these cells. Whether epithelial cells produce a different interferon (from fibroblasts or leukocytes) in response to virus infection, and what functions are affected in such cells by the known interferons should certainly be investigated. Ultimately it is in these cells that those of us interested in viral and malignant disease want to examine the mechanisms involved in the inhibition of viral and cell growth by interferon.

VII PROSPECTS AND PREDICTIONS

It is fairly obvious that basic work on interferons is going to expand enormously. Investigators in widely differing areas of research are going to be interested in studying the actions of interferons *per se*, and in using interferons as tools for elucidating the mechanisms underlying the functions affected by interferons. This will happen whether the clinical use of interferon progresses or not, although the data emerging from basic studies on interferons effects on cell functions may be particularly useful in making decisions about clinical trials as long as supplies are limited. *In vitro* work and even work in animal model systems requires relatively little interferon, and as much information should be got out of these systems as possible.

Some aspects of interferon action are clearly going to be studied intensely. I believe these will include: (1) the interaction with the membrane; (2) how the growth inhibitory stimulus is passed through the membrane and cytoplasm; (3) regulatory effects on the effector cells of the immune system. There will also almost certainly be a concentration of effort on studying the effects of immune interferons. Some areas however may be neglected, and should not be. Among these, I would put the use of animal model tumours (mouse) to investigate the mechanism of the antitumour effect, and the study of interferon action in epithelial cells; the first demands a commitment to producing and purifying large amounts of mouse interferons and the second to culturing real epithelial cells.

There is one area which could be of great interest both scientifically and practically, and that is the effect of interferon on the expression of surface antigens. With monoclonal antibodies available to membrane antigens, which may be tissue or tumour specific, it will be possible to assess quantitatively and directly the effect of interferons on the level of expression of the antigens. It is perhaps not too hopeful to envisage the combined use of interferon and a specific monoclonal antibody (to a tumour surface antigen which is increased by interferon) as being effective therapy against some human tumours.

VIII WHAT SORT OF HORMONE?

The comparison of interferons to hormones has been made now for several years rather vaguely by more than one visionary. We should perhaps ask in a more specific way whether interferon really can be classified in this way. The Oxford English Dictionary gives the definition of a hormone as "a substance formed in an organ and serving to excite some vital process such as secretion". This won't quite do for interferons because their synthesis is not confined to one organ but appears to occur in all manner of cells and tissues. The original Greek word however sounds promising; *ormo*—"to set in motion, to urge on, stir up", and the Homeric word from which it derives, is even better—*ormi*—"an assault, attack, the first shock or onset in war". Interferons certainly stir up and urge on all manner of differentiated functions and quite dramatically present the first assault against virus infection and possibly the growth of malignant cells. I suggest therefore that interferons are Homeric hormones; heroic molecules which, like true heroes, start the fight and draw others with them. In 1980 it looks as though these molecules, perhaps when used with other agents, might under the right circumstances actually win some battles. Even if this turns out not to be the case they will certainly help us to define and understand the nature of the adversary.

IX REFERENCES

Adams, A., Strander, H. and Cantell, K. (1975). *J. gen. Virol.* **28**, 207–217.
Aguet, M. (1980). *Nature* **284**, 459–461.
Allfreid, L. E. and Porter, K. R. (1979). *In* "Surfaces of Normal and malignant cells" (Ed. R. O. Hynes), pp. 21–54. John Wiley, Chichester.
Andersson, J., Gronvik, K. O., Larsson, E. L. and Coutinho, A. (1979). *Eur. J. Immunol.* **9**, 581–587.
Ankel, H., Chany, C., Galliot, B., Chevalier, J. and Robert, M. (1973). *Proc. natn. Acad. Sci. U.S.A.* **70**, 2360–2363.
Attallah, A. M., Needy, C. F., Noguchi, P. D. and Ellsberg, B. L. (1979) *Int. J. Cancer* **24,** 49–52.
Attallah, A. M., Fleisher, J. R., Neefe, A., Kazakis, A., Noguchi, P. D. (1980). Proceedings of Conference on the Regulatory Functions of Interferons. New York. Oct. 1979. *Proc natn. Acad. Sci. U.S.A.* in press.
Baglioni, C. (1979). *Cell* **17**, 255–264.
Balkwill, F. R. (1979). *Cancer Immunol. Immunother.* **7**, 7–14.
Balkwill, F. R. and Taylor-Papadimitriou, J. (1978). *Nature* **274**, 798–800.

Balkwill, F. R. Watling, D., Taylor-Papadimitriou, J. (1978). *Int. J. Cancer.* **22**, 258–265.
Beck, G., Poindron, P., Illinger, D., Beck, J. P., Ebel, J. P. and Falcoff, R. (1974). *FEBS Letters* **48**, 297–300.
Bernheim, J. L., Dorian, R. E. and Mendelsohn, J. (1978). *J. Immunol.* **120**, 955–965.
Besançon, F. and Ankel, H. (1974). *Nature* **252**, 478–480.
Billiau, A., Sobis, H. and De Somer, P. (1973). *Int. J. Cancer* **12**, 646–653.
Blalock, J. E. and Stanton, J. D. (1980). *Nature* **283**, 406–408.
Bourgeade, M. F. and Chany, C. (1976). *Proc. Soc. exp. Biol. Med.* **153**, 501–504.
Bourgeade, M. F., Chany, C., Merigan, T. C. (1980). *J. gen. Virol.* **46**, 449–454.
Brouty-Boye, D. and Tovey, M. G. (1978). *Intervirology* **9**, 243–244.
Brown, K. D., Freidkin, M. and Rozengurt, E. (1980). *Proc. natn. Acad. Sci. U.S.A.* in press.
Calvet, M-C. and Gresser, I. (1979). *Nature* **278**, 558–560.
Ceriani, R. L., Taylor-Papadimitriou, J., Peterson, J. A. and Brown, P. A. (1979). *In vitro* **15**, 356–360.
Chang, E. H., Mims, S. J., Triche, T. J. and Friedman, R. M. (1977). *J. gen. Virol.* **34**, 363–367.
Chang, E. H., Jay, E. T. and Friedman, R. M. (1978). *Proc. natn. Acad. Sci. U.S.A.* **75**, 1859–1863.
Chany, C. (1976). *Biomedicine* **24**, 148–157.
Chany, C., Gregoire, A., Vignal, M., Lemaitre-Moncuitt, J., Brown, P., Besancon, F., Suarez, H. and Cassingena, R. (1973). *Proc. natn. Acad. Sci. U.S.A.* **70**, 557–561.
Chany, C., Vignal, M., Couillin, P., Van Cong, N., Boue, J. and Boue, A. (1975). *Proc. natn. Acad. Sci. U.S.A.* **72**, 3129–3133.
Chany, C., Rousset, S., Bourgeade, M. F., Mathieu, D. and Gregoire, A. (1980). *Proc. natn. Acad. Sci.* in press.
Collyn-d'Hooghe, M., Brouty-Boye, D., Malaise, E. P. and Gresser, I. (1977). *Exp. Cell Res.* **105**, 73–75.
Coutinho, A., Larsson, E. L., Gronvik, K. O. and Andersson, J. (1979). *Eur. J. Immunol.* **9**, 587–592.
De Clercq, E., Edy, V. G. and Cassiman, J. J. (1975). *Nature* **256**, 132–134.
De Maeyer, E., De Maeyer-Guignard, J. (1977). *Tex. Rep. Biol. Med.* **35**, 370–380.
Dianzani, F., Zucca, M., Scuphan, A. and Georgiades, J. A. (1980). *Nature* **283**, 400–403.
Donahoe, R. M. and Huang, K. Y. (1976). *Infect. Immunol.* **13**, 1250–1256.
Eichhorn, J. H. and Peterkofsky, B. (1979). *J. Cell Biol.* **82**, 572–576.
Einhorn, S. and Strander, H. (1977). *J. gen. Virol.* **35**, 573–580.
Epstein, L. B., Lee, S. H. S. and Epstein, C. J. (1980). *Cell Immunol.* **50**, 191–194.
Farrell, P. J., Balkow, K., Hunt, T. and Jackson, R. (1977). *Cell* **11**, 187–200.
Folkman, J. and Moscona, A. (1978). *Nature* **273**, 345–349.
Fournier, F., Falcoff, E. and Chany, C. (1967). *J. Immunol.* **99**, 1036–1041.
Frayssinet, C., Gresser, I., Tovey, M. and Lindahl, P. (1973). *Nature* **245**, 146–147.
Friedkin, M., Legg, A. and Rozengurt, E. (1979). *Proc. natn. Acad. Sci. U.S.A.* **76**, 3909–3912.
Friedman, R. M. and Pastan, I. (1969). *Biochem. biophys. Res. Commun.* **36**, 735–740.
Friedman, R. M. and Ramseur, J. M. (1974). *Proc. natn. Acad. Sci. U.S.A.* **71**, 3542–3544.
Friedman, R. M. (1977). *Bact. Rev.* **41**, 543–567.
Gisler, R. H., Lindahl, P. and Gresser, I. (1974). *J. Immunol.* **113**, 438–444.
Gospodarowicz, D. and Moran, J. S. (1976). *A. Rev. Biochem.* **45**, 531–558.

Greaves, M. F. and Janossy, G. (1972). *Transplant Rev.* **11**, 87–130.
Green, H. (1978). *Cell* **15**, 801–811.
Greenberg, H. B., Pollard, R. B., Lutwick, L. I., Gregory, P. B., Robinson, W. S. and Merigan, T. C. (1976). *New Engl. J. Med.* **295**, 517–522.
Gresser, I. (1977). *Cell Immunol.* **34**, 406–415.
Gresser, I. and Bourali-Maury, C. (1973). *Proc. Soc. exp. Biol. Med.* **144**, 896–899.
Gresser, I., Brouty-Boye, D., Thomas, M. T. and Macieira-Coelho, A. (1970). *Proc. natn. Acad. Sci. U.S.A.* **66**, 1052–1057.
Gresser, I. and Tovey, M. G. (1978). *Biochim. biophys. Acta* **516**, 231–247.
Gresser, I., De Maeyer-Guignard, J., Tovey, M. G. and De Maeyer, E. (1979). *Proc. natn. Acad. Sci. U.S.A.* **76**, 5308–5312.
Gresser, I., Maury, C. and Brouty-Boye, D. (1972). *Nature* **239**, 167–168.
Gresser, I., Thomas, T., Brouty-Boye, D. and Maceira-Coelho, A. (1971). *Proc. Soc. exp. Biol. Med.* **137**, 1258–1261.
Gresser, I., Tovey, M. G., Maury, C., Chouroulinkov, I. (1975). *Nature* **258**, 76–78.
Grollman, E. F., Lee, G., Ramos, S., Lazo, P. S., Kaback, R., Friedman, R. and Kohn, L. D. (1978). *Cancer Res.* **38**, 4172–4185.
Grossberg, S. and Keary, S. (1980). *Proc. natn. Acad. Sci. U.S.A.* in press.
Hollta, E., Pohjanpelto, P. and Janne, J. (1979). *FEBS Letters* **97**, 9–14.
Hovanessian, A. G., Wood, J., Meurs, E. and Montagnier, L. (1979). *Proc. natn. Acad. Sci. U.S.A.* **76**, 3261–3265.
Huet, C., Gresser, I., Bandu, M. T., and Lindahl, P. (1974). *Proc. Soc. exp. Biol. Med.* **147**, 52–55.
Hynes, R. O. (1976). *Biochim. biophys. Acta* **458**, 73–107.
Hynes, R. O. (1979). In "Surfaces of Normal and Malignant Cells" (Ed. R. O. Hynes), pp. 1–20. John Wiley, Chichester.
Ida, S., Hooks, J. J., Siraganian, R. P. and Notkins, A. I. (1977). *J. exp. Med.* **145**, 892–906.
Illinger, D., Coupin, G., Richards, M. and Poindron, P. (1976). *FEBS Letters* **64**, 391–395.
Isaacs, A. and Lindenmann, J. (1957). *Proc. R. Soc. Lond.* (*Biol*) **147**, 258–267.
Janne, J., Poso, H. and Raina, A. (1978). *Biochim. biophys. Acta* **473**, 241–293.
Kahn, P. and Shin, S. (1979). *J. Cell Biol.* **82**, 1–16.
Kerr, I. and Brown, R. E. (1978). *Proc. natn. Acad. Sci. U.S.A.* **75**, 256–260.
Killander, D., Lindahl, P., Lundin, L., Leary, P. and Gresser, I. (1976). *Eur. J. Immunol.* 56–59.
Kimchi, A., Shure, H. and Revel, M. (1979). *Nature* **282**, 849–851.
Knight, E. and Korant, B. D. (1977). *Biochem. biophys. Res. Comm.* **74**, 707–713.
Kohn, L, D., Friedman, R. M., Holmes, J. M. and Lee, G. (1976). *Proc. natn. Acad. Sci. U.S.A.* **73**, 3695–3699.
Lebleu, B., Sen, G. C., Shaila, S., Cabrer, B. and Lengyel, P. (1976). *Proc. natn. Acad. Sci. U.S.A.* **73**, 3107–3111.
Lee, S. H. S. and Epstein, L. B. (1980). *Cell Immunol.* **50**, 177–190.
Lindahl, P., Leary, P. and Gresser, I. (1972). *Proc natn. Acad. Sci. U.S.A.* **69**, 721–725.
Lindahl, P., Leary, P. and Gresser, I. (1973). *Proc. natn. Acad. Sci.* **70**, 2785–2788.
Lindahl-Magnusson, P., Leary, P. and Gresser, I. (1972). *Nature New Biol.* **237**, 120–121.
Macpherson, I. A. and Montagnier, L. (1964). *Virology* **23**, 291–294.
Maheshwari, R. K., Demsey, A. E., Mohanty, S. B. and Friedman, R. M. (1980). *Proc. natn. Acad. Sci. U.S.A.* in press.

Materese, G. and Rossi, G. (1977). *J. Cell Biol.* **75**, 344–354.
Matsuno, T. and Shirasawa, N. (1978). *Biochim. biophys. Acta* **538**, 188–194.
Matsuyama, M. (1979). *Exp. Cell Res.* **124**, 253–259.
Meldolesi, M. T., Friedman, R. M. and Kohn, L. D. (1977). *Biochem. biophys. Res. Comm.* **79**, 239–246.
Mellstedt, H., Ahre, A., Bjorkholm, M., Holm, G., Johansson, B., Strander, H. (1979) *Lancet,* 245–247.
Merigan, T. C., Sikora, K., Breeden, J. H., Levy, R., Rosenberg, S. A. (1978). *N. Engl. J. Med.* **299**, 1449–1453.
Miller, Z., Lovelace, E., Gallo, M. and Pastan, I. (1975). *Science* **190**, 1213–1215.
Nebert, D. W. and Friedman, R. M. (1973). *J. Virol.* **11**, 193–197.
Nicholson, E. L. (1976). *Biochim. biophys. Acta.* **458**, 1–72.
O'Neill, C. H., Riddle, P. N. and Jordan, P. W. (1979). *Cell* **16**, 909–918.
Pardee, A. B., Dubrow, R., Hamlin, J. and Kletzien, A. (1978). *A. Rev. Biochem.* **47**, 715–750.
Paucker, K., Cantell, K. and Henle, W. (1962). *Virology* **17**, 324–334.
Paucker, K., Dalton, B. J., Ogburn, C. A. and Torma, E. (1975). *Proc. natn. Acad. Sci. U.S.A.* **72**, 4587–4591.
Pfeffer, L. M., Wang, E. and Tamm, I. (1980). *J. Cell Biol.* **85**, 9–17.
Pitha, P. M., Rowe, W. P. and Oxman, M. N. (1976). *Virology* **70**, 324–338.
Perkins, M. E., Ju, T. H. and Hynes, R. O. (1979). *Cell* **16**, 941–952.
Pollack, R., Osborn, M., Weber, K. (1975a). *Proc. natn. Acad. Sci. U.S.A.* **72**, 994–998.
Pollack, R., Risser, R., Conlon, S., Freedman, V., Shin, S. and Rifkin, D. (1975b). *In* "Proteases and Biological Control", pp. 885–889. Cold Spring Harbour, New York.
Raff, M. C., Abney, E., Brocker, J. P. and Hornby-Smith, A. (1978). *Cell* **15**, 813–822.
Reisinger, D. M. and Martin, E. M. (1980). *Proc. natn. Acad. Sci. U.S.A.* in press.
Revel, M., Bash, D. and Ruddle, F. H. (1976). *Nature* **260**, 139–141.
Rheinwald, J. and Green, H. (1975). *Cell* **6**, 331–343.
Riviere, Y., Gresser, I., Guillon, J. C. and Tovey, M. G. (1977). *Proc. natn. Acad. Sci. U.S.A.* **74**, 2135–2139.
Roberts, W. K., Hovanessian, A., Brown, R. E., Clemens, M. J. and Kerr, I. M. (1976). *Nature* **264**, 477–480.
Rozee, K, R., Katz, L. J. and McFarlane, E. S. (1969). *Can. J. Microbiol.* **15**, 969–974.
Rossi, G. B., Dolei, A., Cioe, L., Benedetto, A., Matarese, G. P. and Belardelli, F. (1977a). *Proc. natn. Acad. Sci. U.S.A.* **74**, 2036–2040.
Rossi, G. B., Matarese, G. P., Grapelli, C., Belardelli, F. and Benedetto, A. (1977b). *Nature* **267**, 50–52.
Rozengurt, E. (1979). *In* "Surfaces of Normal and Malignant Cells" (Ed. R. O. Hynes), pp. 323–343. John Wiley, Chichester.
Rozengurt, E., Legg, A. and Pettican, P. (1979). *Proc. natn. Acad. Sci. U.S.A.* **76**, 1284–1287.
Rubin, R. W. and Warren, R. H. (1979). *J. Cell Biol.* **82**, 103–113.
Saksela, E., Timonen, T. and Cantell, K. (1979). *Scand. J. Immunol.* **10**, 257–266.
Schroder, E. W., Chou, I. N., Jaken, S. and Black, P. H. (1978). *Nature* **276**, 828–829.
Senger, D. R., Wirth, D. F. and Hynes, R. O. (1979). *Cell* **16**, 885–893.
Shirasawa, N. and Matsuno, T. (1979). *Biochim. biophys. Acta* **562**, 271–280.
Shimizu, N. and Sokawa, Y. (1979). *J. Biol. Chem.* **254**, 12034–12037.
Slater, D. L., Shulman, L., Lawrence, J. B., Revel, M. and Ruddle, F. H. (1978). *J. Virol.* **25**, 319–325.
Smith, J. A. and Martin, L. (1973). *Proc. natn. Acad. Sci. U.S.A.* **70**, 1263–1267.

Sokawa, Y., Watanabe, Y., Watanabe, Y. and Kawade, Y. (1977). *Nature* **268**, 236–238.

Sreevalson, T., Taylor-Papadimitriou, J. and Rozengurt, E. (1979). *Biochem. biophys. Res. Comm.* **87**, 679–685.

Sreevalson, T., Rozengurt, E., Taylor-Papadimitriou, J. and Burchell, J. (1980). *J. Cell Physiol.* in press.

Steinberg, B. M. and Pollack, R. (1979). *Virology* **99**, 302–311.

Stewart, W. E. II. Gosser, L. B. and Lockhart, R. Z. Jr. (1971). *J. Virol.* **7**, 792–801.

Stewart, W. E. II, De Clercq, E., Billiau, A., Desmyter, J. and De Somer, P. (1972). *Proc. natn. Acad. Sci. U.S.A.* **69**, 1851–1854.

Stoker, M. G. P., Pigott, D. and Taylor-Papadimitriou, J. (1976). *Nature* **264**, 764–767.

Strander, H. and Einhorn, S. (1977). *Int. J. Cancer* **19**, 468–473.

Sutherland, E. W. (1972). *Science* **177**, 401–308.

Tabor, R., Rekosh, D., Baltimore, D. (1971). *J. Virol.* **8**, 395–401.

Tan, Y. H., Tischfield, J. and Ruddle, F. H. (1973). *J. exp. Med.* **137**, 317–330.

Tan, Y. H., Schreider, E. L., Tischfield, J., Epstein, C. J., Ruddle, F. H. (1974). *Science* **186**, 61–63.

Tan, Y. H. (1976). *Nature* **260**, 141–143.

Taylor, J. (1964). *Biochem. biophys. Res. Comm.* **14**, 447–451.

Taylor-Papadimitriou, J. and Fentiman, I. S. (1980). "Commentaries on research in Breast Cancer" (Eds R. D. Bulbrook and J. Taylor), in press. Alan Liss, Washington.

Taylor-Papadimitriou, J., Purkiss, P. and Fentiman, I. S. (1980). *J. Cell Physiol.* **102**, 317–323.

Todaro, G. J. and De Larco, J. E. (1978). *Cancer Res.* **38**, 4147–4154.

Tovey, M. G., Rochette-Egly, C. and Castagna, M. (1979). *Proc. natn. Acad. Sci. U.S.A.* **76**, 3890–3893.

Trinchieri, G., Santoli, D. (1978). *J. exp. Med.* **147**, 1314–1333.

Valle, M. J., Jordon, G. W., Haahr, S. and Merigan, T. C. (1975). *J. Immunol.* **115**, 230–233.

van't Hull, E. V., Schellekens, H., Lowenberg, B. and de Vries, M. (1978). *Cancer Res.* **38**, 911–914.

Vengris, V. C., Stollar, B. D. and Pitha, P. M. (1975). *Virology* **65**, 410–417.

Vengris, V. E., Reynolds, F. H., Hollenberg, M. D. and Pitha, P. M. (1976). *Virology* **72**, 486–493.

Weber, J. M. and Stewart, R. B. (1975). *J. gen. Virol.* **28**, 363–372.

Williams, B. R. G. and Kerr, I. M. (1978). *Nature* **276**, 88–89.

Wood, J. N. and Hovanessian, A. E. (1979). *Nature* **282**, 74–76.

Yaron, M., Yaron, I., Gurani-Rotman, D., Revel, M., Linder, H. R. and Zor, U. (1977). *Nature* **267**, 457–459.

Yau, P. M. P., Godefroy-Colburn, T., Birge, C. H., Ramabhadran, T. U. and Thach, R. E. (1978). *J. Virol.* **27**, 648–658.

Yeatman, T. J. (1980). *Proc. natn. Acad. Sci. U.S.A.* in press.

Younger, J. S. (1977). *Tex. Rep. Biol. Med.* **35**, 17–35.

Zilberstein, A., Federman, P., Shulman, L. and Revel, M. (1976). *FEBS Letters* **68**, 119–124.

The Type I Human Interferon Gene System; Chromosomal Location and Control of Expression

DEREK C. BURKE

Department of Biological Sciences, University of Warwick, Coventry, UK

I INTRODUCTION

There are several reasons for studying the molecular biology of interferon formation. The primary reason is that this system provides a model system to study the induction and repression of a eukaryotic gene, since in response to viruses or double-stranded RNA, a dormant cellular gene is activated, new messenger RNA (mRNA) is produced for a few hours and the system is then switched off completely. Translation of this mRNA produces Type I* interferon, a molecule with a very high antiviral activity, which also affects cell growth and the immune response. Since several interferons have now been purified to homogeneity, and amino acid sequencing is in progress, the products of this gene system are becoming well characterized. However another reason for investigating this system is that interferon has attracted considerable attention as an antiviral and anticancer agent. If it does turn out to be clinically useful, then large amounts of interferon will be needed—produced either by induction of human cells in culture, manipulation of the gene into a bacterial cell or possibly by chemical synthesis. The relevance of increased understanding at the fundamental level to these processes is self-evident.

There are two types of human Type I interferon: these are called α (the major species made by leukocytes) and β (the major species made by fibroblasts) (Stewart *et al.*, 1980). A general outline of the mechanism of interferon formation has been known for some years. Viruses and double-stranded RNAs probably activate the interferon system by a common mechanism: the formation of double-stranded RNA in the cell cytoplasm (Marcus and Sekellick, 1980). Viruses form double-stranded RNA as a by-product of virus replication, while the double-stranded RNAs probably enter the cell intact (Pitha and Hutchinson, 1977). The double-stranded RNA then, either directly or indirectly, triggers the transcription of a cellular gene, producing a messenger RNA, which is subsequently translated; the protein is glycosylated and secreted. However, this scheme, like charity, covers a multitude of sins. We still know very little about the mechanism of activation of the interferon gene, but good progress has been made in understanding the processes that follow gene induction, using new methods in cell biology, somatic cell genetics and molecular biology. It is the purpose of this review to summarize briefly the present situation which has been the central interest of our group for the last five years.

II LOCALIZATION OF THE INTERFERON GENE(S)

A The Interferon Gene is a Nuclear Gene

Early experiments showed that the interferon gene was a cellular gene since treatment of chick, mouse or human cells with low doses of actinomycin D inhibited interferon production. This implied that DNA-directed RNA synthesis was essential for interferon formation and since the inducing virus was an RNA virus, cellular DNA must be essential. This was confirmed by

*Type I interferons are induced by viruses or double-stranded RNAs, Type II interferons by treatment of the immunologically competent cell with the appropriate antigen or by treatment of lymphocytes with mitogens. The two types are quite distinct.

irradiating chick cells with UV light before interferon induction: the capacity to make interferon was lost with single-hit kinetics (see review by Burke, 1966).

More recently, it has been shown that the gene is nuclear by using cell enucleation techniques (Burke and Veomett, 1977). If either mouse or human cells were enucleated by treatment with cytochalasin B followed by centrifugation, then the cells failed to produce interferon, whether they were enucleated either just before or just after induction.

B Chromosomal Localization of the Interferon Gene

Somatic cell hybrids have been widely used for the assignment of genes to particular chromosomes, by making use of the fact that such hybrids preferentially lose chromosomes of one of the fusion partners. Clones of hybrid cells can therefore be selected and characterized and those chromosomes which are essential for a particular gene function identified. Further, since the chromosomal complement of these clones is unstable, it is often possible to derive subclones which have lost further chromosomes, and thus establish a correlation between loss of a particular chromosome and of the gene function being studied. Mouse–human hybrids lose human chromosomes, and can therefore be used to identify the chromosomal location of the human gene, including the human interferon gene. Such assignments need considerable caution in interpretation: cultures of hybrid cells are rarely homogenous and the cultures may consist of two or more populations of cells with different chromosomal complements. Two techniques are available for determining which chromosomes are present in a cell hybrid, karyotyping and isozyme analysis. The former is limited by the fact that only a few cells (e.g. 50) are analysed, with the possibility that minor sub-lines are missed; the latter by the fact that the human chromosome composition that results is the average for the whole culture. Since very small amounts of interferon can readily be detected in the bioassay, the production of a relatively large amount of interferon per cell from a small proportion of the cells could easily be confused with a lower yield from all the cells that are present, thus considerably confusing the gene assignment. In addition, since cell hybrids continuously lose human chromosomes, it is important to determine which human chromosomes are present and whether the cells produce human interferon at the same passage level. Finally, it has become clear that interferon genes can be present in a cell but not expressed, e.g. in Chinese hamster cells (see below), and that such genes may then be expressed in hybrids. If human cells contain such genes it would complicate the analysis considerably.

In initial studies, Tan *et al.* (1974) concluded that two human chromosomes (2, 5) were required for human interferon production. However the interferon titres were low and, because of the factors described above, the result was not conclusive. Morgan and Faik (1977), using a single pair of hybrids, concluded that chromosome 5 only was required. We therefore decided to re-investigate the question by analysing a larger series of hybrids, initially to see whether we could determine whether one or two chromosomes were required, and then use the hybrids for studying the control of interferon formation. Finally, we hoped that some of the hybrids might have lost the control element that switches off the production of interferon, so that such cells might produce either very high yields of interferon or produce interferon over a long period of time.

The two human Type I interferons, α and β, are known to differ in antigenicity and primary structure, so that they are certainly different proteins (Vilček, in preparation). Moreover they are translated from different mRNAs (Cavalieri *et al.*, 1977a), so that there are either two genes for human interferon (one for α and one for β), or else a single gene product is processed in two different ways to produce distinct mRNAs.* We therefore examined hybrids which had both human lymphocytes and human fibroblasts as parents in order to see if the hybrids with different parents produced different types of human interferon. These hybrids were either gifts from colleagues or were made in this laboratory by fusion of human diploid fibroblasts with mouse L-A9 cells or mouse PG 19 cells.

A number of hybrids were then surveyed for their ability to produce mouse and human interferons after induction with NDV strain F. The results (Meager *et al.*, 1979a) showed that the hybrids could be grouped into three classes; those that made high yields of human interferon when compared with parental yield, those that made low yields and those that made no human interferon (Table I). All the hybrids made mouse interferon. The hybrids that made no human interferon clearly either lacked the gene or, if present,

TABLE I Human Interferon Production by Mouse–Human Hybrids

Hybrid	Human interferon yield[a] (1st tested)
CTP 34	830
HL 15	670[b]
HL 53	250[b]
CTP 41	2
HL 20	16[b]
HL 35	4[a]

[a] units/ml/10^6 cells.
[b] The human parent yielded 800 units/ml/10^6 cells.

*Note added in proof: Recent work has shown that the two genes are distinct but structurally related (Taniguchi *et al.*, 1980.)

it was firmly repressed. It was more difficult to interpret the results obtained with the low producers; the small amount of interferon produced could either have been due to a low yield from all the cells or a high yield from a few. Because of this ambiguity, it was decided not to proceed any further with their analysis. When the human chromosomes present in the high producers were determined (Table II), a large number of human chromosomes were

TABLE II Human Chromosomes of Some Mouse–Human Hybrids

Hybrid	Human chromosomes																						
CTP 34[a]		2		4	5	6	7		9			12		14	15	16	(17)[d]	18		20			X
HL 15[a]	1	2			5	6	7		9		11	12		14	15	16	17	18	19	20	21		X
HL 53[a]	1	2			5	(6)	(7)		9	10	11	12			15	16	17	18	19	20		22	X
CTP 41[b]		2				6	7							14	15	16		18		20			X
HL 20[b]		(2)				(6)																	
HL 35[b]	1	2			5						11	12	13	14	15	16		18			21	22	
DUR 4[c]			3		5					10	11	12	13	14			17	18			21	22	X
HOR P9[c]				4						10	11	12		14					19		21	22	X
HL 22[c]					(5)		7				11			14		16	17	18		(20)			

[a] High producers.
[b] Low producers.
[c] Non producers.
[d] Brackets signify that the chromosome is present in less than 10% metaphases or trace isozyme activity.

TABLE III Sensitivities of Human–Mouse Cell Hybrids to Diphtheria Toxin

	IF production and diphtheria toxin sensitivity		
Hybrid	Human IF production	Sensitivity to diphtheria toxin[a]	Presence of chromosome 5[b]
HL 15	+	$1{\cdot}0 \times 10^{-3}$	+
HL 53	+	$1{\cdot}0 \times 10^{-3}$	+
HL 8	−	$2{\cdot}5 \times 10^{-3}$	±
HL 54	−	$3{\cdot}2 \times 10^{-3}$	NT
CTP 34	+	$5{\cdot}0 \times 10^{-3}$	+
HL 60	−	$6{\cdot}3 \times 10^{-3}$	±
DUR 4	−	$6{\cdot}3 \times 10^{-3}$	+
HL 42	±	$1{\cdot}0 \times 10^{-2}$	+
HL 24	−	$2{\cdot}0 \times 10^{-2}$	−
HL 10	−	$5{\cdot}0 \times 10^{-2}$	−
HL 44	−	$6{\cdot}3 \times 10^{-2}$	−

[a] Concentration giving 50% inhibition of protein synthesis.
[b] As determined by karyotyping or isozyme analysis.
NT, not tested.

found to be present, including chromosomes 2 and 5 and also chromosome 9.

Since chromosome 5 had been shown to be important in two previous studies and was present in all our high producers, this chromosome was studied first. Chromosome 5 carries the gene for diphtheria toxin sensitivity and since human cells are very sensitive to diphtheria toxin and mouse cells relatively insensitive, any mouse–human hybrids that grow in the presence of diphtheria toxin must have lost the gene and will have often lost human chromosome 5. Determination of the sensitivity of a number of hybrid clones to diphtheria toxin (Table III) showed that this correlated well with the presence of chromosome 5, but not so well with the capacity to make human interferon. We therefore prepared a series of diphtheria toxin resistant subclones of the high producer CTP 34, determined their capacity to produce human interferon and determined which human chromosomes had been lost

TABLE IV Diphtheria Toxin-resistant Subclones of CTP 34

Subclone	Human IF yield[a]	Human chromosomes lost
Parent	830	—
DTR 1[b]	445	5
2	740	5 15 18
3	106	5
4	21	5 6 (9)[c] 15X
5	0	5(6) 9 15 16X
6	168	5 15
7	0	5 9
8	0	5 9
9	740	5 15 18
SC 4	0	2 9 15 18

[a] Yield/ml/10^6 cells.
[b] DTR, diphtheria toxin resistant; SC, subclone.
[c] Brackets signify that the chromosome is present in less than 10% metaphases or trace isozyme activity.

(Table IV). All the diphtheria toxin-resistant subclones had lost chromosome 5, but they had not all lost the capacity to make human interferon. However it was noticed that the capacity to make human interferon did correlate with human chromosome 9; this was the first piece of evidence for the involvement of chromosome 9.

We also analysed a series of nonselected subclones of HL 15 (Table V) and found again that the loss of chromosome 9 correlated with the loss of interferon production. A similar conclusion was reached by the analysis of a series of subclones of a Chinese hamster–human hybrid, all of which lacked chromosome 2 (Table VI). Thus analysis of the clones and subclones showed that the capacity to make human interferon correlated well with the presence of chromosome 9, but did not correlate well with either chromosomes 2,

TABLE V Subclones of HL 15

Subclone	Human IF yield[a]	Human chromosomes lost
Parent	670	—
SC 9	190	(7)[b]
SC 14	9	1 9 15 20
SC 3a	45	(10)
SC 3b	0	1(5) 7 9(10) 17 18 20 22

[a] units/ml/10^6 cells.
[b] Brackets signify that the chromosome is present in less than 10% metaphases or trace isozyme activity.

TABLE VI Subclones of a Chinese Hamster Hybrid 46.6.1

Subclones	Human IF yield[a]	Chromosomes		
		2	5	9
Parent	135	−	+	+
1	0	−	+	−
2	84	−	+	+
3	230	−	+	+
5	420	−	+	+
7	37	−	+	±
8	375	−	+	+
9	167	−	+	+
10	71	−	+	+

[a] yield/ml/10^6 cells.

5 or 2 and 5 (Table VII). Further analysis of HL 42 and of two Chinese hamster–human hybrids showed (Table VIII) a good correlation between interferon production and the short arm of chromosome 9.

At this point we decided that it would be difficult to establish any firmer correlation by further analysis of subclones and we sought evidence for or against chromosome 9 by another route. We were not able to devise any method for selecting for and against chromosome 9, but it is possible to select for or against chromosome X by growing cells in medium containing hypoxanthine, aminopterin and thymidine (which selects for the presence of hypoxanthine-guanine-phosphoribosyl-transferase (HGPRT), or in medium containing 8-azaguanine (which selects against cells containing HGPRT). By using a naturally occurring translocation, in which chromosomes X and 9 are fused, it is possible in this way to select for and against chromosome 9. Hybrids were therefore made by fusing mouse L-A9 cells with GM 705, a

Table VII Summarized Segregation Analysis of IF and Human Chromosomes 2, 5, 2 and 5 and 9 in 13 Independent Primary Human–Mouse Hybrids and 16 Subclones

Chromosome	Hybrids				Subclones			
	Concordant		Discordant		Concordant		Discordant	
	+ +	− −	+ −	− +	+ +	− −	+ −	− +
2	3	6		4	10	1		5
5	3	6		4	2	3	8	3
2 and 5	3	10[a]		[a]	2	1	8	2
9	3	10			10	6		

\+ + IF present; enzyme marker / chromosome present;
− − IF absent; enzyme marker / chromosome absent;
\+ − IF present; enzyme marker / chromosome absent;
− + IF absent; enzyme marker / chromosome present.

[a] One clone contained both chromosome 5 and chromosome 2 and failed to produce IF; but karyotype analysis indicated that 2 and 5 were present in different cells.

Table VIII Markers on Chromosome 9

Hybrid	Human IF yield[a]	Markers		
		AK_3 (short arm)	$ACON_S$	AK_1 (long arm)
HL 42	9	−		+
Cl 13	140	+	+	+
Cl 23	0	−	−	+

[a] yield/ml/10^6 cells.

Table IX Results of a Fusion Between L-A9 × GM 705 Cells

Hybrid	Human IF yield[a]	Human chromosomes
GLA	125	2 3 5 6 7 8(9) 11 12 14 15 16 18 19 20 21 X X/9
GLB	125	(2)3 6 7 8 11 12 14 15 16 18 19 20 21 X X/9
GLC	0	(2)3 6 7 8 11 14 15 16 18 19 20 21

[a] units/ml/10^6 cells.

human fibroblast carrying an X : 9 translocation. One of these (GL-A, Table IX) which yielded as much human interferon as the human parent (100 units/ml/10^6 cells), was treated with diphtheria toxin to select against chromosome 5 and generate GL-B, which still made human interferon. When GL-B cells were treated with 8-azaguanine to select against the X : 9 chromosome, the hybrid GL-C was produced which had lost X:9, and also the capacity to make human interferon. A similar result was obtained when the mouse melanoma cells PG 19 were used as one parent, with GM 705 as the other (Meager *et al.* 1979b). One of the hybrid clones produced, GP-2, lacked both chromosomes 2 and 5, but had an X : 9 chromosome and made human interferon. It was concluded that chromosome 9, but not chromosomes 2 or 5, was essential for interferon formation.

This result conflicts with the earlier reports of Tan *et al.* (1974) and Morgan and Faik (1977) and also with a recently published paper by Slate and Ruddle (1979) which concluded that either chromosomes 2 or 5 were essential for interferon formation. However none of the hybrids used by Tan *et al.* (1974) or by Slate and Ruddle (1979) contained chromosome 9, and so these data do not exclude an important role for chromosome 9. Since these publications, both Slate and Ruddle and also C. Chany (personal communication) have shown that chromosome 9 contain structural genes for human interferon. Chany also has evidence for the involvement of chromosomes 2 and 5. There is therefore agreement from three groups that chromosome 9 carries an interferon gene, but conflicting evidence over chromosomes 2 and 5; with positive evidence from two groups although our evidence appears to rule them out. If we exclude trivial explanations for this discrepancy, e.g. that the cultures are heterogeneous or contain translocated chromosomes or portions of chromosomes, then the most likely explanation is that there are several genes for human interferon, one on chromosome 9, that is strongly expressed, and others on chromosomes 2 and 5 that are repressed in some hybrids, or may only express in others at a low level (e.g. in our low producers). Two ways to resolve these issues are apparent: the first is to study mouse–human hybrids which contain only a single human chromosome, i.e. 2, 5 or 9, probably translocated onto X, and the other is to examine the genomic DNA from the hybrids by hybridization with a probe from a cloned interferon gene.

III CONTROL OF INTERFERON PRODUCTION IN SOMATIC CELL HYBRIDS

A Mouse–Human Hybrids Produce Human Fibroblast Interferon

Human cells may produce either leukocyte (α) or fibroblast (β) interferon.

or more usually, a mixture of the two (Vilček, in preparation). They can be distinguished by use of specific antisera or by titration on heterologous cells, since α interferon is active on a much wider range of cells than β interferon. Both Meager *et al.* (1979a) and Slate and Ruddle (1979) found that all the hybrids examined produced fibroblast interferon, whether the human parent was either a fibroblast or a lymphocyte, and despite the fact that the fibroblast parent of our hybrids produced a small amount of α interferon in addition to the β interferon when treated with virus (A. Meager, personal communication).

We do not understand what controls whether α or β interferons are formed but it is clear that this control system is tightly switched over to β interferon production in the hybrids. This may reflect the dominant control by the mouse cell since recent amino acid sequencing results with purified mouse (Taira *et al.*, 1980) and human (Knight *et al.*, 1980; Zoon *et al.*, 1980) interferons have shown that the two major components of purified mouse interferon appear to have a common polypeptide chain, differing only in the amount of glycosylation, whose amino acid sequence is related to that of human β interferon. It is only a minor component of mouse interferon (C in the nomenclature of Taira *et al.*, 1980) that has an amino acid sequence related to human α interferon and this interferon has only been found in the interferon made by mouse Erlich ascites cells. This suggests that mouse fibroblast cells make predominantly a "fibroblast-type" interferon, and that this pattern is imposed on the human gene(s) present in the hybrids.

B Repressed Interferon Genes can be Switched On in Hybrids

Guggenheim *et al.* (1968) fused nucleated chick erythrocytes (which cannot produce chick interferon) with two different human cell lines, one able to produce human interferon, the other unable to produce interferon. The heterokaryons formed were then tested for the formation of human and chick interferons: those derived from the interferon-competent human cells were able to produce both human and chick interferons, while those formed from the interferon-defective human cells produced neither interferon. This suggests that human gene(s) could activate the inactive chick interferon gene in the dormant erythrocyte. This result was confirmed and extended by Burke *et al.* (1980), who found that the production of chick interferon by mouse–chick heterokaryons correlated with the reactivation of the chick erythrocyte nucleus, as shown by the appearance of nucleoli and the production of a chick enzyme.

Similar conclusions can be drawn from the study of somatic cell hybrids. Morgan and Faik (1977) found that hybrids formed between Chinese hamster cells, which do not make hamster interferon, and human cells can make both hamster and mouse interferons. Similar results were obtained by Carver *et al.* (1968) using mouse–Syrian hamster hybrids, and by Meager *et al.* (1979a) using Chinese hamster–human hybrids. Vero cells, obtained from the African green monkey, are unable to make interferon but produce small amounts of monkey interferon after fusion with mouse cells (A. Meager, personal communication). These studies suggest that the permissive cells produce some substance that is essential for activation of the interferon gene(s).

C Priming and Superinduction in Cell Hybrids

When cells are treated with low doses of homologous interferon before induction, the subsequent interferon yields are often increased, a phenomenon called priming. Mouse and human cells differ in their priming characteristics and it is therefore possible to determine whether the priming characteristics of the hybrids are those of the mouse or human parents and whether the production of both mouse and human interferons can be primed by pre-treatment of mouse–human hybrids with mouse interferon, or whether only the production of mouse interferon is affected. In other words, does priming affect a process common to both mouse and human genes or not? Graves and Meager (1980) found that production of both interferons were affected by priming with mouse interferon, and that the dose of mouse interferon that gave optimal priming of the mouse interferon production was also optimal for human interferon production. Thus the human gene is treated as if it were a mouse gene as far as priming is concerned.

A similar conclusion was reached as a result of a study of superinduction of interferon production in the hybrids. When cells are induced to produce interferon by treatment with double-stranded RNA, it is possible, using certain dose schedules of cycloheximide and actinomycin to increase the yields of interferon, a phenomenon known as superinduction. The mouse parents of the hybrids used by Meager *et al.* (1979a, b) were either L-A9 cells, which

TABLE X Induction and Superinduction of Mouse–Human Hybrids

	Interferon yield[a]			
	Human		Mouse	
Cell	Induced	Super-induced	Induced	Super-induced
PG 19			130	5100
L-A_9			0	0
HEF	300	6000		
CTP 34	4	280	40	7000
HL 15	0	0	0	0

[a] units/ml/10^6 cells.

do not respond to poly rI : poly rC or superinduce, or PG-19 cells which do respond to poly rI : poly rC and also superinduce. The human parents were either T lymphocytes, which do not respond to poly rI : poly rC or superinduce, or human diploid fibroblasts (HEF) which do respond to poly rI : poly rC and also superinduce. When the hybrids were tested for their ability to respond to poly rI : poly rC or to superinduce, it was found (Table X) that CTP 34, a hybrid of the mouse PG 19 cell and a human T lymphocyte, responded to poly rI : poly rC and superinduced like its mouse parent, producing and superproducing both mouse and human interferons. On the other hand, HL 15, a hybrid of the mouse L-A9 cells and HEF, failed to respond to poly rI : poly rC or superinduce, both the human and mouse genes being completely unresponsive. Thus the hybrids behave like the mouse parent both in their response to poly rI : poly rC and to superinduction.

D Glycosylation of Interferon in Cell Hybrids

The interferon polypeptide is glycosylated by a series of cellular enzymes before secretion and this process can be inhibited by analogues such as 2-deoxyglucose and glucosamine. Since human and mouse interferon production differ in their sensitivity to inhibition by 2-deoxyglucose, human interferon production being considerably more sensitive, it is possible to see whether the two interferons produced by mouse–human hybrids behave similarly or not in their sensitivity to 2-deoxyglucose. T. Mason and A. Meager (personal communication) found that both interferons showed the sensitivity characteristic of mouse interferon production—showing that the glycosylation of both interferons is characteristic of the mouse parent.

Thus in every respect so far investigated the hybrids behave like the mouse parent, suggesting that the control systems examined so far—for the production, priming, responsiveness to poly rI : poly rC, superinduction and glycosylation—are under mouse genetic control. The human interferon produced by these hybrids is human only in respect of its amino acid sequence, which determines the species specificity, but otherwise it is a mouse cell product.

IV CONTROL OF TRANSCRIPTION OF THE HUMAN INTERFERON GENE(S)

A Control of Transcription in Superinduction

The superinduction of interferon yields by the appropriate addition of cycloheximide and actinomycin has usually been interpreted by suggesting that there are two distinct mechanisms controlling interferon production. One controls the transcription of the interferon mRNA, and the other controls the translational activity of the mRNA once it is formed, probably by prolonging the half-life of the mRNA (Stewart, 1979a). Although there is evidence that both control systems operate in human cells, it is likely that superinduction is mainly controlled by the second mechanism.

When cells are superinduced the kinetics of interferon production are changed. Although the initial rate of interferon production is unaffected, interferon production continues for very much longer (Fig. 1). Interferon mRNA is translated faithfully after micro-injection into *Xenopus* oocytes to

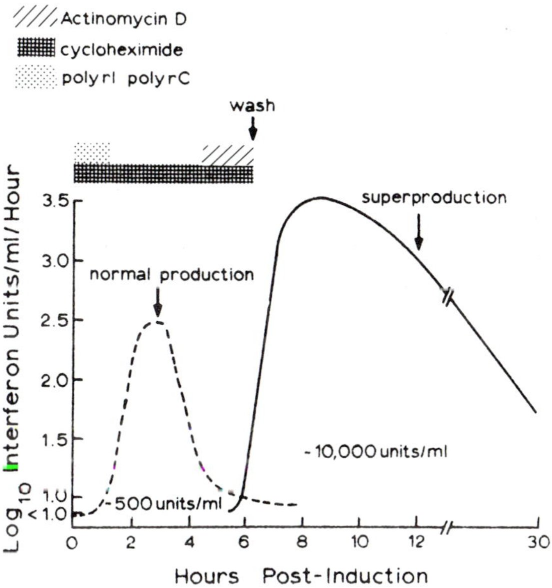

Fig. 1 Superproduction of interferon. The system illustrated is the human fibroblast method described by Havell and Vilček (1972) from Stewart (1979a).

produce biologically active material, and this assay can be used to estimate the amount of interferon mRNA present in the cells (Stewart, 1979b). Application of this technique showed that there was more interferon mRNA present in superinduced cells than in control cells at about 6 h after induction (Raj and Pitha, 1977; Sehgal *et al.*, 1977; Cavalieri *et al.*, 1977b). This suggests that the earlier cessation of interferon production in control cells is due to inactivation or degradation of the interferon mRNA by a process which was considerably slower in superinduced cells. Cavalieri *et al.* (1977b) also found that addition of cycloheximide alone caused prolonged transcription of the interferon mRNA as well as decreased inactivation or degradation.

In summary, there are probably at least three ways by which the amount of interferon produced can be regulated at the transcriptional level:

(i) By an increased rate of transcription of the gene, occurring possibly with cycloheximide and certainly with BUdR and sodium butyrate (see below).
(ii) By increasing the half-life of the mRNA.
(iii) By increasing the translatability of the message that is formed. e.g. by interferon mRNA competing more efficiently in translation (Garry and Waite, 1979).

B Increased Rate of Transcription after Treatment with 5-Bromodeoxyuridine

Many transformed B-lymphocytes—such as those derived from patients infected with Epstein-Barr virus or Burkitt's lymphoma—produce good yields of leukocyte interferon after induction with Sendai virus (Strander *et al.*, 1975). Tovey *et al.* 1977 found that pretreatment of the Namalwa line of lymphoblastoid cells with 5-bromodeoxyuridine (BUdR) led to increased yields of interferon after induction with Sendai virus. BUdR affects cells by at least two mechanisms—by a process that requires incorporation of the analogue into cellular DNA, such as the induction of C-type viruses and one that does not require incorporation but affects specialized gene function,

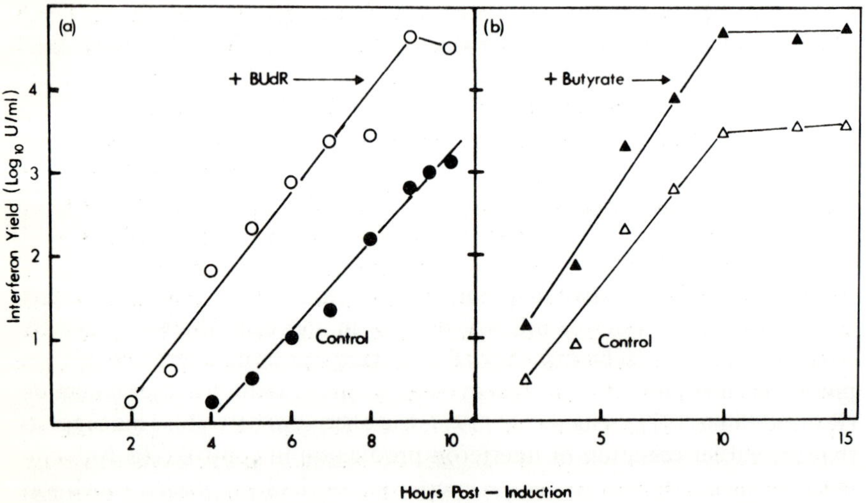

Fig. 2 Rate of production of interferon in: (a) control and BUdR-treated Namalwa cells after induction with Sendai virus; (b) control and sodium butyrate-treated Namalwa cells after induction with Sendai virus.

e.g. in differentiation. The latter is reversed by addition of deoxycytidine since the effect of the analogue appears to be on the enzyme ribonucleotide reductase. Thus BUdR can cause either gene activation or gene repression. The increase in interferon yield is not reversed by addition of deoxycytidine, and does require incorporation of the analogue into cellular DNA (Baker *et al.*, 1979). Further, since pretreatment with BUdR leads to an increased rate of synthesis of interferon (Fig. 2), the effect is quite different from the superinduction phenomenon. These facts suggest that BUdR is acting by a gene activation mechanism, and J. Shuttleworth and J. Morser (personal communication) have recently shown in this laboratory that BUdR pretreatment increases the rate of interferon mRNA production, although it has no effect on the half-life of the mRNA. Thus BUdR increases the yield of interferon by increasing the rate of transcription, although the mechanism is unknown.

C Increased Rate of Transcription after Treatment with Sodium Butyrate

Pretreatment of Namalwa cells with 1 mM sodium butyrate also increases the yield after induction with Sendai virus (Johnston, 1979; Adolf and Swetley, 1979) because of an increase in the rate of interferon production (Fig. 2*b*) (Baker *et al.*, 1980). Butyrate has been widely studied as an activator of transcription and it has a number of effects on cells. It is not known how these effects are related, i.e. which is causal and which is consequential, but all the effects described in the literature have been found in butyrate-treated Namalwa cells (Baker *et al.*, 1980). These include inhibition of DNA synthesis and of cell division, blockage of the cell cycle in G_1, slowing of the rates of RNA and protein synthesis and increased acetylation of histones. Since at least 36 h pretreatment with sodium butyrate is needed to get the maximum stimulation, it is unlikely that the events which occur rapidly, such as the inhibition of DNA synthesis and of cell division and the increased acetylation of histones, are the direct causes of the increased interferon production. It is more likely that one of the more slowly acting effects, such as the effect on RNA synthesis, is responsible. Direct measurement of the amount of interferon mRNA by the *Xenopus* oocyte inoculation technique has shown a substantial increase in the rate of interferon mRNA synthesis, without any effect on the half-life of the mRNA (Morser *et al.*, 1980). Thus sodium butyrate, like BUdR causes an increase in interferon yield by increasing the rate of transcription of interferon mRNA. The two agents clearly work in different ways since their effect on cell metabolism is quite distinct. They act synergistically on interferon production too, interferon production being higher when both reagents are used than when either is used separately (J. Shuttleworth and J. Morser, personal communication).

V TRANSLATION OF HUMAN INTERFERON mRNA

A In Cell-free Systems

There have been several reports of the translation of human fibroblast interferon mRNA in cell-free systems (Reynolds and Pitha, 1975; Pestka *et al.*, 1975; Reynolds *et al.*, 1975) with the production of low titres of biologically active material. The systems are however much less efficient (about 500-fold) than is injection into *Xenopus* oocytes, and it is possible that the cell-free system produces a polypeptide precursor to fibroblast interferon which has little or no biological activity. There is some evidence for this (Pestka *et al.*, 1977), and Weissenbach *et al.* (1979) have shown that when an antiserum prepared against human fibroblast interferon is added to the products of the cell-free system, a single polypeptide of 23 000 molecular weight is precipitated, which is possibly the precursor. Recently a rather similar conclusion was reached during a study of leukocyte interferon formation in Namalwa cells (Morser and Colman, 1981). Addition of inhibitors of proteolysis stops interferon formation, probably as a result of inhibition of a post-translational cleavage mechanism.

B In *Xenopus* Oocytes

Oocytes are able to carry out a number of post-translational processes such as glycosylation, polypeptide cleavage, acetylation and phosphorylation and they will in addition continue to translate injected mRNAs for long periods. It is therefore not surprising that human interferon mRNAs are translated much more efficiently in oocytes than in cell-free systems and the system has been used by a number of workers, not only to study the mechanism of translation but more commonly to assay interferon mRNA levels in, for example, normal and superinduced cells, and during the purification of interferon mRNA for cloning (Morser *et al.*, 1979). However it was surprising to find that the leukocyte interferon, formed by translation of the injected message, was actively secreted from the oocytes, and appeared in the surrounding medium (Colman and Morser, 1979). This secretion was not due to leakage from the oocyte, since when globin mRNA was coinjected with the interferon mRNA, the interferon was secreted but the globin was not. The leukocyte mRNA had a long half-life, synthesis and secretion of the product occurring at a constant rate for at least 5 days (J. Morser and A. Colman, personal communication). A survey of the fate of the products obtained when a large number of different mRNAs were injected into *Xenopus* oocytes showed that every secretable protein was secreted from the oocyte (Lane *et al.*, 1980). Thus the oocyte treats the translation product in exactly the same way as does the cell from which the message came; the newly synthesized polypeptide is associated with a membrane, probably by means of a hydrophobic leader sequence, is there glycosylated, while the membrane becomes part of a secretory granule before leaving the cell (Colman *et al.*, 1980).

VI PROSPECTS

This brief review shows that substantial progress has been made in understanding the events following activation of the interferon gene, and future work will fill out details, particularly as cloned interferon genes become available as hybridization probes (Nagata *et al.*, 1980). We still know little however of the processes that link the inducer (double-stranded RNA?) with gene derepression. This has always been the hardest area to probe. It is also the most interesting, and here too the availability of cloned genes should help. It should not now be difficult to clone, and thereby to sequence, the genome DNA of the interferon gene. It is an article of faith with molecular biologists that when such an inducible gene as interferon is sequenced somewhere, probably upstream from the 5′ end, will be a sequence that controls inducibility.

VII ACKNOWLEDGEMENTS

I am much indebted to my colleagues Dr Tony Meager, Dr Alan Morris and Dr John Morser for many hours of stimulatory discussions and for their criticisms of this manuscript.

VIII REFERENCES

Adolf, G. R. and Swetly, P. (1979). *Virology* **99**, 158–166.
Baker, P. N., Bradshaw, T. K., Morser, J. and Burke, D. C. (1979). *J. gen. Virol.* **45**, 177–184.
Baker, P. N., Morser, J. and Burke, D. C. (1980). *J. Interferon Res.* **1**, in press.
Burke, D. C. (1966). *In* "Interferons" (Ed. N. B. Finter), pp. 55–86. North-Holland, Amsterdam.
Burke, D. C. and Veomett, G. (1977). *Proc. natn. Acad. Sci. U.S.A.* **74**, 3391–3395.
Burke, D. C., Ege, T. and Ringertz, N. R. (1980). *J. gen. Virol.* in press.
Carver, D. H., Seto, D. S. Y. and Midgeon, B. R. (1968). *Science* **160**, 558–564.
Cavalieri, R. L., Havell, E. A., Vilček, J. and Pestka, S. (1977a). *Proc. natn. Acad. Sci. U.S.A.* **74**, 3287–3291.
Cavalieri, R. L., Havell, E. A., Vilček, J. and Pestka, S. (1977b). *Proc. natn. Acad. Sci. U.S.A.* **74**, 4415–4419.
Colman, A. and Morser, J. (1979). *Cell* **17**, 517–526.
Colman, A., Lane, C., Craig, R., Boulton, A., Mohun, T. and Morser, J. (1980). *Eur. J. Biochem.* in press.
Garry, R. F. and Waite, M. R. F. (1979). *Virology* **96**, 121–128.
Graves, H. E. and Meager, A. (1980). *J. gen. Virol.* **47**, 489–495.
Guggenheim, M. A., Friedman, R. M. and Rabson, A. S. (1968). *Science* **159**, 542–543.
Havell, E. A. and Vilček, J. (1972). *Antimicrob. Agents Chemother.* **2**, 476–484.

Johnston, M. D. (1979). Europatent 520. Wellcome Foundation.

Knight, E. Jr., Hunkapiller, M. W., Korant, B. D., Hardy, R. W. F. and Hood, L. E. (1980). *Science* **207**, 525–526.

Lane, C. D., Colman, A., Mohun, T., Morser, J., Champion, J., Kourides, I., Craig, R., Higgins, S., James, T. C., Appelbaum, S. W., Ohlsson, R. I., Paucha, E., Houghton, M., Matthews, J. and Miflin, B. J. (1980). *Eur. J. Biochem.* in press.

Marcus, P. I. and Sekellick, M. J. (1980). *J. gen. Virol.* **47**, 89–96.

Meager, A., Graves, H. E., Walker, J. R., Burke, D. C., Swallow, D. M. and Westerwald, A. (1979a). *J. gen. Virol.* **45**, 309–321.

Meager, A., Graves, H., Burke, D. C. and Swallow, D. M. (1979b). *Nature* **280**, 493–495.

Morgan, M. J. and Faik, P. (1977). *Brit. J. Cancer* **36**, 254.

Morser, J. and Colman, A. (1981). *J. gen. Virol.* in press.

Morser, J., Flint, J., Meager, A., Graves, H., Baker, P. N., Colman, A. and Burke, D. C. (1979). *J. gen. Virol.* **44**, 231–234.

Morser, J., Meager, A. and Colman, A. (1980). *FEBS Letters* in press.

Nagata, S., Taira, H., Hall, A., Johnsrud, L., Streuli, M., Ecsödi, J., Boll, W., Cantell, K. and Weissman, C. (1980). *Nature, London* **284**, 316–320.

Pestka, S., McInnes, J., Havell, E. A. and Vilček, J. (1975). *Proc. natn. Acad. Sci. U.S.A.* **72**, 3898–3906.

Pestka, S., McInnes, J., Weiss, D., Havell, E. A. and Vilček, J. (1977). *Ann. N.Y. Acad. Sci.* **284**, 697–720.

Pitha, P. M. and Hutchinson, D. W. (1977). *In* "Interferons and their Actions" (Ed. W. E. Stewart, II), pp. 13–35. CRC Press, Cleveland, Ohio.

Raj, N. B. K. and Pitha, P. M. (1977). *Proc. natn. Acad. Sci. U.S.A.* **74**, 1483–1487.

Reynolds, F. H., Jr and Pitha, P. M. (1975). *Biochem. biophys. Res. Commun.* **65**, 107–114.

Reynolds, F. H., Jr Premkumar, E. and Pitha, P. M. (1975). *Proc. natn. Acad. Sci. U.S.A.* **72**, 4881–4887.

Sehgal, P. B., Dobberstein, B. and Tamm, I. (1977). *Proc. natn. Acad. Sci. U.S.A.* **74**, 3409–3413.

Slate, D. L. and Ruddle, F. H. (1979). *Cell* **16**, 171–180.

Stewart II, W. E. (1979a). *In* "The Interferon System", pp. 97–103. Springer, Vien and New York.

Stewart II, W. E. (1979b). *In* "The Interferon System", pp. 93–95. Springer, Vien and New York.

Stewart II, W. E., Blalock, J. E., Burke, D. C., Chany, C., Dunnick, J. K., Falcoff, E., Friedman, R. M., Golano, G. J., Joklik, W. K., Vilček, J. T., Youngner, J. S. and Zoon, K. C. (1980). *Nature* **286**, 110.

Strander, H., Mogenson, K. E. and Cantell, K. (1975). *J. clin. Microbiol.* **1**, 116–124.

Taira, H., Broeze, R. J., Jayaram, B. M., Lengyel, P., Hunkapiller, M. W. and Hood, L. E. (1980). *Science* **207**, 528–530.

Tan, Y. H., Creagan, R. P. and Ruddle, F. M. (1974). *Proc. natn. Acad. Sci. U.S.A.* **71**, 2251–2255.

Taniguchi, T., Mantei, N., Schwarzstein, M., Nogota, S., Muramatsu, M. and Weissmann, C. (1980). *Nature* **285**, 547–549.

Tovey, M. G., Begon-Lours, J., Gresser, I. and Morris, A. G. (1977). *Nature, London* **267**, 455–456.

Weissenbach, J., Zeevi, M., Landau, T. and Revel, M. (1979). *Eur. J. Biochem.* **98**, 1–8.

Zoon, K. C., Smith, M. E., Bridgen, P. J., Anfinsen, C. B., Hunkapiller, M. W. and Hood, L. E. (1980). *Science* **207**, 527–528.

The Purity and Safety of Interferons Prepared for Clinical Use: The Case for Lymphoblastoid Interferon

N. B. FINTER AND K. H. FANTES

Wellcome Research Laboratories, Langley Court, Beckenham, Kent, UK

I INTRODUCTION

There is no question that, ideally, an interferon preparation intended for clinical use should consist only of interferon molecules suspended in a menstruum of known and acceptable composition. In the future this ideal may be achieved with interferons (or possibly smaller related proteins with interferon activity) made in large amounts by genetic engineering techniques, or by chemical synthesis, and purified to homogeneity (though whether such products, possibly lacking particular sugar moieties present in native interferons will nevertheless have the same behaviour *in vivo* is a matter for debate and ultimately for clinical verification). At the present time, the interferon in the preparations used in clinical medicine has for the most part represented 1% or even less by weight of the total and uncharacterized proteins present. Our colleagues engaged in the development of pharmaceutical products have expressed incredulity and derision at the concept that a drug intended for repeated use in man should be so impure. Yet in our experience, a 600 litre culture of crude lymphoblastoid interferon may contain only 10–50 mg of interferon protein in the presence of 2–3 kg of other proteins. Since our purification procedures involve significant losses, it is no small feat to achieve purification of the final interferon preparations even to the level of 1%. In practice, we have routinely obtained lymphoblastoid interferon of considerably higher purity with a specific activity of greater than 10^7 units/mg protein, and not infrequently approaching 10^8. We have however usually added human serum albumin at 1–3 mg/ml to the final purified preparations, as this marginally improves their stability. The Sephadex profile of one of our routine batches is shown in Fig. 1.

Purification problems and losses are found with other types of interferon, and so there has had to be a compromise between making material of a very high purity and having sufficient material to treat patients. It is therefore necessary to consider what impurities may be present in particular interferon preparations, and to decide what restrictions or limits should be imposed on them. In other words, what consequences may follow their injection on a single occasion and after repeated administration? Various side-effects have been noted to follow the use of interferon in patients, namely pyrexia, lassitude, malaise, leukopenia and occasionally other effects such as hypotension, etc. (Merigan, 1977). These effects have sometimes set a limit to the amounts of interferon which could be given or to the duration of treatment. Some of these effects may reflect intrinsic activities of interferon but others the consequences of contaminants in particular preparations. We would emphasize that what is at issue is the nature and quantity of the contaminants in the interferon preparation as intended for clinical use. There are precedents for the use of less than ideal starting materials in the production or manufacture of medicinal products, and for example insulin is made from pancreases collected from abattoirs. Thus, although human buffy coat leukocytes are, from the quality control point of view, far from ideal as a source of interferon, what matters is the safety of the interferon made from them. Incidentally, although crude buffy coat interferon was at one time used in man and without any serious consequences, we believe that few would now contemplate the administration of this or any other unpurified interferon.

The heterogeneity of interferon poses further problems. For example, leukocyte-type interferon derived from buffy coat cells contains two principal molecular species with weights of approximately 21 000 and 15 000 daltons,

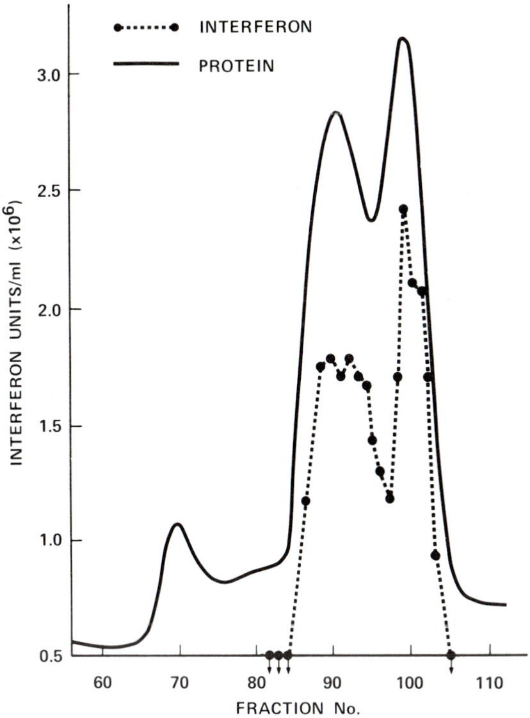

Fig. 1 Analysis carried out by Dr G. Allen on Sephadex G 75 of a routine batch of our interferon which has been used in patients. The two peaks of protein and interferon activity have been found in all our preparations. There is a small amount of protein of higher molecular weight. The specific activity of this particular preparation (before adding stabilizer) was 0·88 $\times 10^8$ international units/mg total protein. Protein markers suggested approximate molecular weights of 22 000 and 18 500 for the two interferon peaks.

and differing in their biological properties (Stewart and Desmyter, 1975; Stewart, 1979). It is not known whether one of these species may be preferable for particular clinical purposes, or indeed if they differ in their effects. Also, different methods of induction and purification may selectively enrich the final preparation with one or the other species. Crude leukocyte-type interferon derived from Namalwa cells is contaminated with an appreciable amount of interferon with the antigenic specificity characteristic of fibroblast interferon. Clearly, it cannot be assumed that all preparations, e.g. of leukocyte-type interferon, will be identical in their behaviour if they have been prepared in different laboratories and processed by different procedures.

II SOURCES OF INTERFERON FOR CLINICAL USE

Before considering further the extraneous substances which may be present in current preparations of interferon, we will outline how these preparations are made.

A Human Leukocyte Interferon

Until recently, most of the interferon used for clinical purposes has been derived from white blood cells. Cantell and his associates have played the major role in developing this system, and have described their techniques in detail (Cantell *et al.*, 1974; Cantell and Hirvonen, 1977). In brief, the white cell layer ("buffy coat") is separated from donated blood, and contaminating red cells are lysed with ammonium chloride. The pooled white cells from 5–25 donations are washed, resuspended in medium containing "agamma" (i.e. treated with ammonium sulphate) human serum and induced to form interferon by the addition of Sendai virus. After overnight incubation, the cell suspension is centrifuged, and the supernatant contains the crude interferon. This is purified by precipitation with KSCN and extraction of the precipitate with acid aqueous ethanol. The resultant purified interferon (P–IF) contains $0{\cdot}5 \times 10^6 - 1{\cdot}0 \times 10^6$ million international units/mg total protein.

B Human Fibroblast Interferon

Human diploid fibroblasts, particularly certain strains such as FS 4, produce large amounts of interferon when stimulated with the synthetic double-stranded RNA, poly rI: poly rC and treated with the metabolic inhibitors, actinomycin D and cycloheximide, under the so-called superinduction conditions (Havell and Vilček, 1972; Billiau *et al.*, 1973). Such human fibroblast interferon differs in its antigenic specificity, chemical composition and biological properties from the leukocyte-type interferons derived from buffy coat or lymphoblastoid cells.

C Human Lymphoblastoid Interferon

When interferons, and especially preparations made from buffy coat cells, have been used in patients with virus infections or with tumours, some encouraging clinical results have been noted (Baron and Dianzani, 1977; Strander, 1977), but the relatively small amounts available have so far made it very difficult to carry out controlled trials with adequate numbers of patients. In 1974 we therefore decided to explore the use of transformed cells for making interferon, since we felt that if interferon proved useful in medicine, buffy coat cells could not provide enough for widespread clinical use; it would be essential to use cells that can grow in suspension in large tanks. We knew that even the idea of using such cells was heretical, but we reasoned that if the resulting interferon was sufficiently purified and shown to be safe, it would probably be accepted for clinical use, even if initially only for seriously ill patients. With our colleagues, we therefore explored various possibilities including HeLa cells. Within a few months, we saw the data of Strander and colleagues (1975), showing that some human lymphoblastoid cell lines, particularly one termed "Namalwa" could yield substantial amounts of interferon. We soon confirmed their findings, and after studying some 200 lymphoblastoid lines (Christofinis *et al.*, 1980) we decided to establish production of Namalwa interferon on a relatively large scale.

It has long been supposed by most virologists that transformed cells could not be used as a substrate for the production of vaccines or other biologicals. It was said (or believed) that "they"—meaning, of course, the Control Authorities in various countries—would never permit their use, because of the consequences, real or theoretical, which might follow. This dogma became firmly established without actually being put to the test, and precedents from animal medicine were ignored: e.g. millions of cattle have been successfully immunized against foot-and-mouth disease virus with a vaccine made in the BHK line of transformed hamster kidney cells. In fact as Dr Harry Meyer, Director of the Bureau of Biologics, has pointed out (Meyer, 1979), there never was a formal ban on the use of transformed cells—at least in the USA: whether a particular transformed cell line should be used for production depends on the merit of the case, and in particular on the possible risks and potential benefits that might result.

Although several other groups have now followed suit, our decision to make Namalwa cell interferon for clinical purposes was regarded as a folly by most people at the time when we began our studies in 1975. Nevertheless, we went on with our plans and in 1978 we completed the construction of a pilot plant. This is based on a 1000 litre vessel, in which we can grow Namalwa cells in suspension for periods of months at a time. The cells are cultured in medium RPMI 1640 which is supplemented with 7% gamma-irradiated calf serum. As required, 300–500 litre quantities of cells are transferred to a 600 litre production vessel, and treated with sodium butyrate (1–3 mM) for 2–3 d; this substantially increases the subsequent yields of interferon (Johnston, 1979). The cells are induced to form interferon by the addition of Sendai virus, and after overnight incubation the contents of the production vessel are passed through a series of filters ending with one with a pore size of 0·22 μm so that every cell is removed. The filtrate containing the interferon is passed to a hold tank. Under our conditions the yields of interferon per cell are appreciably smaller than those obtained from smaller laboratory cultures, but because of the large batch sizes, substantial total amounts of crude interferon can be obtained. The interferon is passed in line through various purification steps, and the final highly purified material is piped into a sterile suite for the final stages in purification and dispensing. One of the sequences we have used involves precipitation with trichloroacetic acid (Fantes, 1966), treatment with organic solvents (Fantes, 1970) and antibody affinity chromatography (Anfinsen *et al.*, 1974), essentially as described by Bridgen *et al.* (1977) and Zoon *et al.* (1979), and this has yielded material which has been approved for clinical trials in the UK. Based on our experience with this pilot plant, we have now developed much larger production facilities. Part of the fermenter hall from a plant making interferon is shown in Fig. 2.

III THE PROBLEMS WITH NAMALWA CELL INTERFERON

Lymphoblastoid cell lines can be derived from white cells cultured from the blood of most individuals. The cells may transform spontaneously if the donor has been infected with Epstein–Barr (EB) virus, or they may be transformed by the deliberate addition of EB virus. The major objection to cells of the Namalwa lymphoblastoid line is that they originated from a small Ugandan girl who ultimately died from a Burkitt lymphoma. They contain EB virus genome, and the evidence suggests very strongly that the presence of this is responsible for their stably transformed nature. Does this EB virus represent a human tumour virus? Certainly this possibility, which is discussed in detail below, is one which we could not afford to ignore. We have therefore developed techniques for purifying to a very high degree the crude interferon harvested from stimulated Namalwa cell cultures. Because of our preoccupation with the need to satisfy, first, ourselves and subsequently, others with the purity and safety of our product, we have considered very carefully what impurities and contaminants might be present in our crude and final interferon preparations, and what their effects might be. We have also taken into account such theoretical risks as the possible presence of an as yet unidentified oncogenic virus, or a slow virus, or a nucleic acid derived from such an agent. We have therefore not only looked for likely contaminants in our final interferon preparations; we have also deliberately added to crude interferon preparations marker substances, related to possible contaminants but more easily quantitated, and followed their inactivation or elimination during our purification procedures. These markers are listed in Table I, and the following comments can be made.

Fig. 2 (*see opposite*) 1000, 2000 and 4000 litre tanks in a commercial fermentation plant producing lymphoblastoid interferon.

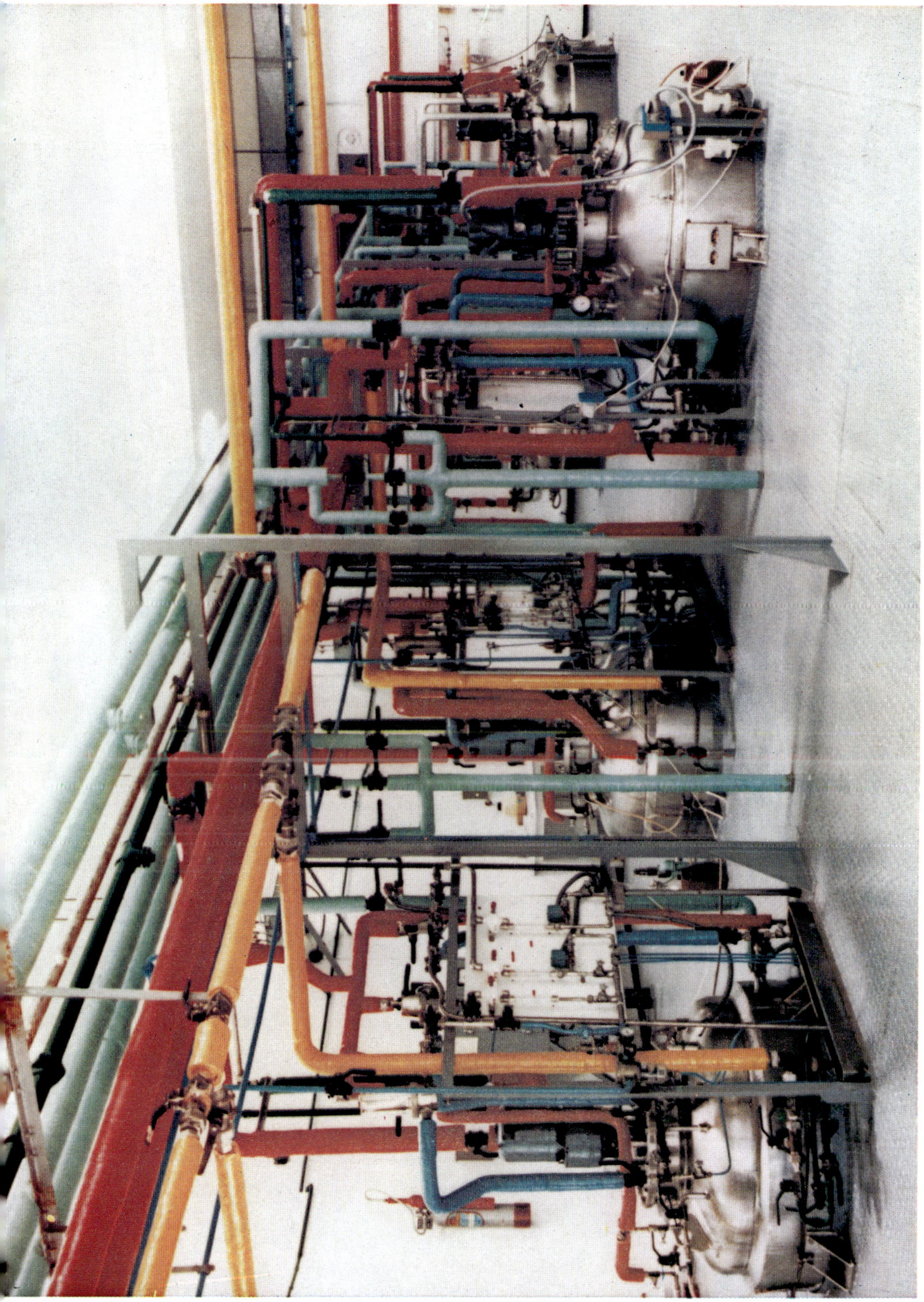

TABLE I Effects of our Purification Procedures Applied to Namalwa Cell Interferon: Inactivation or Elimination of Marker Substances

	Marker added	Minimum amount inactivated or eliminated[a]	Notes
1. Viruses			
animal	Polyoma	7 log p.f.u.	*b*
	Mouse cytomegalo	5·1	*b*
	Canine hepatitis	7·7	*b*
	Cat herpes	4·8	*c*
	Polio type 1	8·4	*c*
	Newcastle disease	11·3 log EID_{50}	
	Sendai	7·8	
	Avian leukosis	6·8 log f.f.u.	*d*
bacterial	Phage T3	9·5 log p.f.u.	*e*
	W31	8·6	*e*
	BF23	11.3	*e*
	ØX174	11·5	*f*
	1-fil	6·7	*f*
	MS2	10·2	*g*
2. Mycoplasmas			
	M. orale	8·8 log c.f.u.	
	M. gallisepticum	8·6	
3. Other infectious agent	Scrapie agent	7 log mouse LD_{50}	
4 Nucleic acid	Polyoma DNA	3·8 log p.f.u.	*b*
	EB virus DNA	385 500 c.p.m.	
	Raji cell DNA	7 095 500 c.p.m.	
5. Bacterial lipopoly-saccharide	*E. coli* endotoxin	99.97%	*h*

[a] None of the added markers was detected in the final purified interferon fraction (except for 0·032% of the added bacterial endotoxin). The values shown thus denote the minimum extent of destruction or inactivation after allowance for the concentration of the interferon during processing.

[b] Validity of results uncertain, since human interferon had some activity in the assay cells used.

[c] Virus added to a dummy serum-containing medium to avoid effects of interferon on assay system.

[d] Rous sarcoma virus (Schmidt-Ruppin strain): virus growth assessed by the COFAL technique.

[e] Containing double-stranded DNA.

[f] Containing single-stranded DNA.

[g] Containing single-stranded RNA.

[h] 100 μg added to 1 litre dummy interferon; 32 ng measured in final fraction equivalent to purified interferon.

A Viruses

Technical problems make it difficult to use, as markers, human viruses such as cytomegalovirus, EB and herpes simplex, etc. which would be most relevant. First, some of these do not grow to high titre, and so only relatively small amounts could be added to the crude interferon: even if none were to be found in the final preparation, this would only indicate elimination of a correspondingly small amount during purification. Second, the antiviral activity in a purified and concentrated interferon preparation would make it difficult to detect residual amounts of a virus which must be grown in human or monkey cells. Even if the cells used can be derived from other animals, the cross-species antiviral activity may be sufficient to make detection difficult, even if this is only 0·1% of the homologous activity in human cells. Before we appreciated this fully, we carried out some studies with animal viruses as shown in Table I. However, our definitive studies were carried out with Sendai, NDV and Rous sarcoma viruses which grow in avian cells (where the human interferon has no activity) and, particularly, with bacterial viruses. Our colleague, Dr Stealey, has studied phages representative of every class in terms of morphology and nucleic acid composition: all were destroyed to the limit of detection, and with most, this represented a loss of 10^{8}–10^{10} p.f.u./ml.

B Nucleic Acids

Dr J. Pagano, Chapel Hill University, North Carolina, USA, kindly provided us with heavily radio-labelled DNA derived from Raji cells (another line of lymphoblastoid cells) and from EB virus. When these were used as markers in our interferon purification procedure, no radioactivity above background level was found in the final purified interferon fraction.

C Scrapie Agent

We used this agent as a representative "slow" virus. In studies in collaboration with Dr G. D. Hunter and colleagues, Agriculture Research Council, Compton, Berkshire, high titre preparations of the agent were added to crude interferon, which was then processed. None was detected in the final interferon fraction.

D Endotoxin

Fever is usually observed after administration of interferon, and sometimes patients suffer rigors. It is important to be sure that such effects are not due to contamination of the preparations with bacterial endotoxin. It was thus reassuring to find that large amounts of deliberately added endotoxin were eliminated during our purification process.

IV IMPURITIES IN INTERFERON PREPARATIONS INTENDED FOR CLINICAL USE

A virus vaccine, made like interferon from cultured mammalian cells, is likely to be given only once or twice in an individual's lifetime. In contrast, an interferon preparation may be administered repeatedly, perhaps once or twice a week for a year or even longer. The presence of impurities in the preparation could have considerable immunological and other consequences and so a very much higher standard of purity is necessary for an interferon preparation than for such a vaccine.

The extraneous substances which may be found in interferon preparations can be considered in three groups. First, there are contaminants of the crude interferon, which come from the cells, culture medium, or the inducer, or are chemicals used in the induction system, or added to increase the yields of interferon. Second, there are whatever reagents are used to purify the interferon, and the buffers, stabilizers, cryoprotective agents, etc. which may be added to the final interferon. Third, at any stage in its manufacture, an interferon preparation may be accidentally contaminated with micro-organisms or other substances. This particular problem will not be considered further because it is one common to the manufacture of vaccines and other biologicals. There are well established production rules which aim to minimize the occurrence of such contaminants, and statutory procedures for testing for them. For example material from the final containers must be tested for bacteriological sterility, for freedom from abnormal toxicity in animals, etc. Such general safety tests applied to interferon preparations will also pick up acutely noxious contaminants.

A Contaminants Derived from the Cells

The cells which are used as the source of interferon are also an obvious potential source of micro-organismal and protein contaminants. Various steps can be taken to minimize the chances that these will be present in the crude interferon, and to remove them from the final product.

With Namalwa cells, a Master Cell Bank can be laid down in liquid nitrogen, and samples can be fully tested by standard techniques for the presence of contaminating bacteria, mycoplasmas and viruses. Cells for production can then be derived from this Master Cell Bank in the same general way as when diploid fibroblasts are used in the production of live polio or rubella virus vaccines. When we tested cells from our Master Cell Bank for infectious agents, we did not detect any, and except for possible accidental contamination, our production cells are also free from these. Since production is carried out within steel tanks linked by steam-sterilized pipes, the chances of contamination are small and, for example, bacterial infection has been infrequent despite the complexity of the plant. A Master Cell Bank can similarly be set up for a diploid fibroblast cell strain used to make interferon (although some strains such as WI-38 and MRC-5 are "clean", it cannot be assumed that others will be). In contrast, every new batch of pooled buffy coat cells is an unknown quantity, and it is not practical to apply the same detailed quality control procedures as are used when testing a Master Cell Bank. From time to time, some of the white cells will be excreting cytomegalovirus, or EB virus, or some other virus such as measles or herpes simplex.

As mentioned, we had to consider that Namalwa cells may be contaminated with an oncogenic agent, either EB virus or some other. Most individuals in all countries are infected with EB virus at some stage in their life, and in the vast majority without clinical symptoms. Did the particular strain in the child, Namalwa, differ significantly from other strains? This question cannot be answered. Certainly, the EB virus present in Namalwa lymphoblastoid cells is different in one important way from most strains in that only about half of the total genome is present (Pritchett *et al.*, 1976), and thus no infectious virus can be formed. Nevertheless, all the cells contain the virus gene or genes which give them their transformed character, and they grow to form tumours when injected into immunosuppressed mice (Nilsson *et al.*, 1977). It is however important to note that disrupted Namalwa cells do not form tumours (J. Garrett, personal communication). Because our interferon passes through four separate 0.22 μm filters during its purification, there cannot be any intact Namalwa cells in our final product. Nevertheless do Namalwa cells when they die release EB virus nucleic acid which might be capable of producing tumours?

In further experiments with Dr Pagano, we therefore looked for EB virus DNA in crude Namalwa cell interferon. A sample of crude interferon contained 40 million international units and a total of 1·5 mg of DNA. When part of this was tested for its content of EB virus DNA by molecular hybridization, none was detected. Considering that the weight of the total cellular DNA in a single Namalwa cell is about 4×10^{12} daltons, and that of the EB virus DNA in a Namalwa cell about 10^8 daltons, we calculated that at most about $0{\cdot}25 \times 10^{-4}$ of the DNA released from Namalwa cells will be represented by EB virus DNA. On this basis our sample contained not more than about 9×10^{-4} μg EB virus DNA/million units of interferon. However, in the experiments already cited, we found that radio-labelled EB virus DNA and cellular DNA were eliminated to the limits of detection from the final interferon fraction by our purification procedures. This of course does not mean that not a single molecule will ever come through the process. However, on the basis of the recovery of interferon activity during purification and the data above, we can calculate that the *maximum* likely amount of EB virus DNA in our final purified interferon will be less than about 0·8 pg/million units of final product, an amount which of course is far too small to be directly measured. Transmission of genetic information to a cell in a recipient, i.e. transfection, would require the EB virus genome to enter that cell and integrate with its DNA. Experience with other herpes viruses has shown that the efficiency of transfection is extremely low, and DNA corresponding to 10^3–10^5 virions is required to transfect a single cell.

It can be argued that Namalwa cells may contain some other oncogenic agent or virus. Our results suggest that any such would also be eliminated by our purification procedures. Also, no C-type virus particles are seen in sections of Namalwa cells, and no reverse transcriptase activity can be detected (P. Baker, personal communication).

There is of course no way in which absolute safety can be guaranteed for interferon made from Namalwa cells but the chances that the product will cause tumours in a recipient must be very small indeed. Risks of a similar magnitude are already accepted in relation to other products and procedures used in medicine, and indeed risks of considerably greater magnitude are part of everyday life. It should also be pointed out that oncogenic viruses could conceivably be present in particular lines of fibroblasts or in some batches of buffy coat cells, and the latter could also be contaminated on occasions with circulating neoplastic cells from an unsuspected primary tumour.

Theoretically, any cells providing interferon might harbour a slow virus such as the agent of progressive multifocal leuko-encephalopathy (the same problem applies to other biologicals and for example it is known that the agent of scrapie contaminated some batches of an arbovirus vaccine derived from infected sheep brains, and used in Scotland to protect sheep against the tick-borne encephalitis, Louping Ill). We know of no evidence to suggest that such an agent is indeed present in Namalwa cells; even if one was, our data on the elimination of deliberately added Scrapie agent during our purification process suggest that it would not be a hazard. To our knowledge no similar assurance has been provided for any other biological.

The cell substrate will also add other contaminants to a crude interferon preparation. White blood cells release endogenous pyrogen, and the presence of this in buffy coat interferon may contribute to the fever that frequently follows its administration (Kauppinen *et al.*, 1977). It is possible that endogenous pyrogen is also released from Namalwa cells (T. Priestman, personal communication). Some reports suggest that there is less fever with fibroblast interferon (Scott *et al.*, 1977; Billiau *et al.*, 1980) but it is not clear whether this reflects absence of endogenous pyrogen from the preparations, or the very low levels of circulating interferon that follow their injection.

Other substances with pharmacological or immunological activity may be generated during the induction process, and for example, Yaron *et al.* (1977) claimed that prostaglandins are produced during interferon formation. Buffy coat cells produce lymphokines, and indeed some of the activities of crude leukocyte interferon have been attributed to their presence, though to our knowledge, without any convincing evidence. We looked for Macrophage Migration Inhibitory Factor in crude Namalwa cell interferon and found none. Immunoglobulin may be released from B lymphocytes and from lymphoblastoid cells, but we have been unable to measure any in our crude interferon. Cells may release histocompatibility antigens, and if the cells are derived from a Master Cell Bank, these will be the same in every interferon preparation. It appears however that Namalwa cells express these antigens very poorly (which unfortunately has made them unattractive to those who have wished to use our waste cells as a source for purifying them).

Dying cells will release various cellular proteins, including lysosomal enzymes, and in consequence, appreciable quantities of ribonuclease are found in crude leukocyte interferon. This enzyme is still detectable in the purified fraction, P-IF which has been used much in clinical work (Winchurch *et al.*, 1977). Namalwa cells grow in culture rather than merely survive, and possibly for this reason crude Namalwa interferon contains much less ribonuclease: none could be detected in our purified preparations (Karpetsky *et al.*, 1979). Other cellular proteins must contaminate all crude interferons, and represent some of the residual impurities in the purified preparation. Biochemical data from one laboratory showed the presence of fibronectin in their purified fibroblast interferon (Billiau *et al.*, 1979).

B Contaminants Derived from the Medium

To make any type of human interferon, it is at present essential to have some human or animal serum in the medium, or at least a serum fraction, if high yields are to be obtained. If untreated human serum is used, there must be the possibility that hepatitis B virus may contaminate the crude interferon, even if the sera have been screened by a sensitive technique, such as radio-immunoassay. No other tests for circulating viruses are applied routinely to donor blood. When interferon is made from diploid fibroblasts or Namalwa cells, calf or pig serum has usually been used in the growth medium. In our production system we have used calf serum which has been irradiated to an extent shown to destroy deliberately added viruses, mycoplasmas and bacteria. Residual calf serum protein in the final product might sensitize the recipient, or cause allergic reactions in an individual already sensitized. Using very sensitive methods including radio-immunoassay and sensitized guinea pigs we have found small amounts of calf protein in our final preparations, but we believe these are not big enough to cause problems; certainly individuals injected repeatedly with our interferon daily for a period of a month have not developed detectable levels of antibodies to the calf proteins. Parenthetically, we would add that although from many points of view, we would dearly like to exclude all calf serum from our culture, we cannot at present do this. On an experimental scale we have used various replacements for serum, including serum albumin, tryptose phosphate broth and enzymatic digests of meat products, but we do not yet have one that is satisfactory and also acceptable from the quality control point of view. It is of course not possible to use hundreds of litres of human serum instead of animal serum.

A point to bear in mind is that if any antibiotics are added to the medium, suitable ones must be chosen, and for example, penicillin should not be used at any stage. Equally any antifoam agent added to the production medium must be acceptable for injection into humans.

C The Inducer and Contaminants from the Inducer Preparation

Both leukocyte and Namalwa interferons are made by adding to the production cells a virus such as Sendai or Newcastle disease, grown in fertile hens' eggs. The crude interferon thus contains not only this virus but also egg proteins and any avian viruses latent in the eggs. It seems very undesirable that a tumour virus, such as avian leukosis virus, should be present in the final interferon preparation. Treatment at pH 2 even for several days does not always destroy viruses, and for example by blind passage, we were able to detect trace amounts of residual infectious virus after treating Sendai virus and Newcastle disease virus at pH 2 for 1–2 days. However, we have shown destruction of these viruses and of Rous sarcoma virus by our purification procedure.

When unpurified buffy coat interferon preparations were used in patients, antibodies to virus and egg proteins were formed in the recipients, though this caused no apparent clinical problems. It thus seems very unlikely that there will be difficulties with the more highly purified preparations now being made in Finland or with our Namalwa cell interferon.

Traces of the double-stranded polyribonucleotide inducer could conceivably be present in fibroblast interferon preparations, but they are likely to be degraded by the nucleases present in human serum.

D Chemicals Used to Increase Interferon Yields

If fibroblast interferon is made by the superinduction procedure, traces of the carcinogen, actinomycin D, and of the toxic chemical, cycloheximide, may be present in the crude interferon. It seems doubtful that any significant amounts will be present in purified preparations, but no evidence on this point has been published. Various chemicals have been used to increase yields of Namalwa cell interferon, and some of these, for example phorbol ester (Adolf and Swetly, 1980) and bromodeoxyuridine (Tovey *et al.*, 1977), are carcinogens. We have treated the cells with sodium butyrate (Johnston, 1979), which significantly increases the yields of interferon; this substance is of course well known in the food industry and presents no toxicological problems.

E Chemicals used in the Purification

These chemicals may be present in the final interferon, and for example, our purified interferon can contain up to 10–15% ethanol, which is removed if the product is freeze-dried. Other chemicals used to purify interferons may also have pharmacological properties; e.g. potassium thiocyanate is used to purify leukocyte interferon, but the final amounts in the P-IF fraction are probably very small. If antibody affinity chromatography is used, the possibility must be considered that some immuno-absorbent will contaminate the product, and this is not just a theoretical problem, based on experience in our laboratories with other products. Other chromatographic materials may similarly get into the product. Concanavalin A used for the chromatographic purification of fibroblast interferon has been found in the product: this substance is both a mitogen and antigenic, and it seems undesirable it should be present in the final preparation. Blue dextran provides a very efficient means for purifying human fibroblast interferon, but it is a carcinogen and must not contaminate an interferon preparation intended for clinical use.

V CONCLUDING REMARKS

Based on what has been said above, we can summarize quite briefly our thoughts on the purity of interferon preparations intended for clinical use. The substrate or ingredients used to make the interferon are not of paramount importance. Even if less than ideal from one or other point of view, their use may be permissible if they confer a significant manufacturing advantage or if there is no reasonable alternative, and provided that the safety of the final product is established beyond reasonable doubt. High purity can be achieved routinely in the production of interferon (see Fig. 1) and the risks, real or imaginary which could result from contaminants in crude interferons should be eliminated by appropriate purification procedures. The efficacy of these should be monitored, if necessary with appropriate marker substances. We do not intend to suggest that interferon preparations of existing types made from leukocytes and fibroblasts may not be perfectly acceptable for clinical use—the control authority in each country will here make its own decision—and certainly such preparations have been of inestimable value in helping to assess the value of interferon in medicine. With larger scale and commercial production, higher standards may be needed, and our experience suggests that these are not impossible to achieve.

VI REFERENCES

Adolf, G. R. and Swetly, P. (1980). *J. gen. Virol.* in press.

Anfinsen, C. B., Bose, S., Corley, L. and Gurari-Rotman, D. (1974). *Proc. natn. Acad. Sci. U.S.A.* **71**, 3139–3142.

Baron, S. and Dianzani, F., Eds (1977). *Tex. Rep. Biol. Med.* **35**, 436–477.

Billiau, A., Joniau, M. and De Somer, P. (1973). *J. gen. Virol.* **19**, 1–8.

Billiau, A., Van Damme, J., Van Leuven, F., Edy, V. G., De Ley, M., Cassiman, J., Van Den Berghe, H. and De Somer, P. (1979). *Antimicrob. Agents Chemother.* **16**, 49–55.

Billiau, A., Heine, J. W., Van Damme, J., Heremans, H. and De Somer, P. (1980). *Ann. N.Y. Acad. Sci.* in press.

Bridgen, P. J., Anfinsen, C. B., Corley, L., Bose, S., Zoon, K. C., Ruegg, V. T. and Buckler, C. E. (1977). *J. biol. Chem.* **252**, 6585–6587.

Cantell, K. and Hirvonen, S. (1977). *Tex. Rep. Biol. Med.* **35**, 138–144.

Cantell, K., Hirvonen, S., Mogensen, K. E. and Pyhala, L. (1974). *In* "In Vitro Monograph" Vol. 3, pp. 35–38.

Christofinis, G., Steel, C. M. and Finter, N. B. (1980). *J. gen. Virol.* in press.

Fantes, K. H. (1966). *In* "Interferons" (Ed. N. B. Finter) pp. 119–180. North-Holland, Amsterdam.

Fantes, K. H. (1970). *Ann. N.Y. Acad. Sci.* **173**, 118–121.

Havell, E. A. and Vilček, J. (1972). *Antimicrob. Agents Chemother.* **2**, 476–484.

Johnston, M. D. (1979). Europatent 520. Wellcome Foundation.

Karpetsky, T. P., Winchurch, R. A., Burman, C. J. and Fantes, K. H. (1979). *J. gen. Virol.* **44**, 241–244.

Kauppinen, H-L., Myllyla, G. and Cantell, K. (1977). *Adv. exp. Med. Biol.* **110**, 1–13.

Merigan, T. C. (1977). *Tex. Rep. Biol. Med.* **35**, 541–547.

Meyer, H. M. (1979). *Adv. exp. Med. Biol.* **118**, 1–5.

Nilsson, K., Giovanella, B. C., Stehlin, J. S. and Klein, G. (1977). *Int. J. Cancer* **19**, 337–344.

Pritchett, R., Pedersen, M. and Kieff, E. (1976). *Virology* **74**, 227–231.

Scott, G. M., Butler, J. K., Cartwright, T., Richards, B. M., Kingham, J. G., Wright, R. and Tyrrell, D. A. J. (1977). *Lancet* **ii**, 402–403.

Stewart II, W. E. (1979). "The Interferon System", pp. 171–183. Springer, New York.

Stewart II, W. E. and Desmyter, J. (1975). *Virology* **67**, 68–78.

Strander, H. (1977). *Tex. Rep. Biol. Med.* **35**, 429–435.

Strander, H. Mogensen, K. E. and Cantell, K. (1975). *J. clin. Microbiol.* **1**, 116–124.

Tovey, M. G., Begon-Lours, J., Gresser, I., Morris, A. G. (1977). *Nature* **267**, 455–456.

Winchurch, R. A., Karpetsky, T. P., Levy, C. C. and Cantell, K. (1977). *J. Virol.* **21**, 1247–1259.

Yaron, M., Yaron, I., Gurari-Rotman, D., Revel, M., Lindner, H. R. and Zor, U. (1977). *Nature* **267**, 457.

Zoon, K. C., Smith, M. E., Bridgen, P. J., Zur Nedden, D. and Anfinsen C. B. (1979). *Proc. natn. Acad. Sci. U.S.A.* **76**, 5601–5605.

Lymphokines, Cytokines and Interferon(s)

STANLEY COHEN AND PIERLUIGI E. BIGAZZI
Department of Pathology, University of Connecticut Health Center, Farmington, Connecticut, USA

> What's in a name? That which we call a rose
> by any other name would smell as sweet.
>
> *William Shakespeare*

I INTRODUCTION

Lymphokines are nonantibody mediator substances produced by appropriately activated lymphocytes. They have diverse biologic effects, including alterations of cell motility, activation of inflammatory cells and induction of cellular proliferation. In addition, certain lymphokines can exert toxic effects on a variety of normal and abnormal target cells. Finally lymphokines exert profound regulatory control of the immune system itself. There are "helper" factors that enhance the capacity of B lymphocytes to produce antibody. In addition, there are "suppressor" factors that diminish B cell reactivity. Under most circumstances, the lymphokines are produced as a "package", i.e. multiple lymphokine activities appear simultaneously. Nevertheless, under appropriate experimental conditions, it is possible to demonstrate restrictions in the range of biologic activity, and these reproducible restrictions suggest that the activities are due to discrete molecular species.

Similarly, it has been found possible to separate different activities by physicochemical manipulations. Thus, even though 90 or so lymphokine activities have been described (Waksman, 1979), it seems clear that these are not 90 distinct entities. There appears to be a smaller set of discrete basic mediators or "mother factors". The apparent diversity of biologic behaviour is a consequence of limitation of the *in vitro* biologic assays used for detection. An additional complication is that these factors are effective in nanogram amounts, and when produced in the laboratory are invariably contaminated by many other products of cellular metabolism and catabolism, often present in significantly higher concentrations than the lymphokines themselves.

Interferon, discovered in 1957 (Isaacs and Lindenmann, 1957), was originally defined in the same way as were the various lymphokines; namely, in terms of an *in vitro* assay system. It was observed that supernatants from cultures of chick chorioallantoic membrane exposed to heat-inactivated influenza virus were capable of conferring protection against live virus. Since those early observations, a large variety of other biologic activities have been ascribed to interferon, many of which mimic those of various lymphokines. This will be discussed in detail below. At this point, however, it should be noted that several years after the original discovery of interferon, Wheelock (1965) reported that mitogen-stimulated lymphocytes could produce interferon. Certain differences from virus-induced interferon led to a distinction between "Type I" or classical interferon and "Type II", or immune interferon. By definition, Type II interferon is a lymphokine.

Meanwhile, the definition of "lymphokine" was undergoing extension. These factors were originally thought to be exclusively T lymphocyte products. In 1973, we demonstrated that B, as well as T cells, could make Migration Inhibition Factor (MIF) (Yoshida *et al.*, 1973). This capacity of B cells to perform a function previously thought unique to T cells was confirmed for MIF and several other lymphokines in many other laboratories (reviewed in Rosenstreich and Wahl, 1979). At about the same time, two groups (Tubergen *et al.*, 1972; Papageorgiou *et al.*, 1972) demonstrated that various established nonlymphoid cell lines could spontaneously release factors with MIF-like activity into the culture medium. Shortly thereafter, our own group reported that virus infection of nonlymphoid cells could trigger the production of soluble mediators with a variety of lymphokine activities (reviewed in Bigazzi, 1979). These factors were termed "cytokines". Thus, on the one hand, as stated above, nonviral activation of lymphoid cells can give rise to a substance or substances similar to or identical with "interferon", as well as lymphokines. On the other hand, viral activation of nonlymphoid cells can give rise to substances similar to various lymphokines as well as interferon. Surprisingly, the implication of this curious symmetry involving factors, defined for the most part operationally, has been largely ignored. In this chapter we will examine the possibility that, just as there are a smaller number of discrete lymphokines than originally thought, there may be more "interferons" than is generally now appreciated. Many of their nonantiviral effects may be due to discrete molecular species identical to or related to the previously described cytokines.

II NONANTIVIRAL EFFECTS OF INTERFERON

This subject has been recently reviewed in great detail (Epstein, 1979). The brief overview that follows is largely patterned after her review. Since this is primarily a speculative essay, we will merely describe some of the findings relating to the nonantiviral effects of interferon, with only minimal reference to specific investigations or investigators. Full documentation and citations may be found in Epstein (1979).

In general, the effects described are biologically assayable activities found in culture supernatants. When a given effect has been ascribed to interferon, it means that the following criteria have been met: (1) the factor responsible for the effect responds to various physicochemical procedures in a manner parallel to that responsible for the antiviral activity; (2) the intensity of the effect parallels increases in antiviral activity during purification procedures, (3) the effect can be abrogated by anti-interferon antisera where available.

A Effects on the Immune System

An enormous body of work on effects of interferon on the immune system has been reported. Both suppressing and enhancing effects of interferon preparations have been described (see Sonnenfeld, 1980). With respect to primary immune responses *in vitro*, low doses of interferon enhance, whereas larger doses suppress plaque-forming responses. Similar findings have been described in *in vivo* studies. Although these results involve IgG and IgM responses, recent reports have focused on IgE-mediated reactions as well. Thus, when murine spleen cells known to synthesize IgE were treated with interferon, their ability to sensitize rat skin *in vivo* for anaphylaxis was inhibited (Ngan *et al.*, 1976).

Interferon preparations can suppress lymphocyte proliferative responses, as has been reported by many laboratories. Interestingly, Miorner *et al.* (1978) found that in the presence of low doses of mitogen, low doses of interferon could enhance blastogenesis. Interferon can enhance cytotoxicity reactions, and enhance the expression of various H-2 antigens on murine lymphoid cells. Interferon can inhibit cutaneous delayed-type hypersensitivity in the mouse (De Maeyer *et al.*, 1975).

Interferon preparations have also been found capable of enhancing macrophage phagocytosis (Donohoe and Huang, 1973), the transformation of monocytes to macrophages (Lee and Epstein, 1978) and production of release of lysosomal enzyme activity. In addition, interferon enhances the tumouricidal activity of macrophages (Schultz *et al.*, 1977). Indeed, the whole catalogue of effects of interferon on macrophages (Schultz, 1980) is almost identical with that describing the effects of lymphokines on macrophages (Adelman *et al.*, 1979).

For the most part the above studies have made use of Type I interferon. A more limited number of studies have demonstrated that Type II interferon has similar immunoregulatory properties.

B Nonimmune Effects.

Interferon can inhibit the growth of a variety of normal and tumour cells (Gresser, 1977). In addition, it can inhibit cell motility in culture (Brouty-Boye and Zetter, 1980). This latter effect has been noted using bovine capillary endothelial cells and skin fibroblasts as targets. Another effect of interferon is its ability to stimulate hyaluronic acid production and prostaglandin synthesis by synovial fibroblasts (Yaron *et al.*, 1976; 1977). A number of studies by Salvin and his associates have shown that interferon preparations have antitumour, antibacterial and antifungal activity. The underlying biochemical mechanisms for these effects have not been elucidated.

An intriguing nonimmunologic, nonantiviral effect of interferon is known as "priming". Small amounts of interferon produced by only a few cells in response to early viral infection may prime many other cells for an enhanced response. Although the mechanism of priming is not fully elucidated, its overall biologic effect is paralleled in the lymphokine system where antigen triggers small numbers of specifically sensitized cells to produce lymphokines. One such lymphokine mediator is a mitogenic factor than can induce additional lymphokine production by the cells present that were not specifically sensitized to the test antigen.

C General Considerations

To summarize this section, the various nonantiviral effects of interferon preparations that have been described fall into one of three categories. (1) They can exert growth regulatory effects, largely by influencing proliferative events in a variety of cell types. Some of the effects on the immune system are probably due to this. (2) They can effect the migration properties of various cell types; this has been studied in only a limited way, and with respect to migration inhibition. We are aware of no studies of possible chemotactic properties of interferons. (3) They can affect the ability of cells to produce characteristic products. Examples cited above include the synthesis of hyaluronic acid and prostaglandin by fibroblasts, the production of various classes of immunoglobulin by immunocytes, and the production and/or release of lysosomal enzymes by macrophages.

In addition, interferon preparations probably enhance inflammatory responses, at least with regard to their antifungal and antitumour activity. There is little direct evidence for this phlogistic effect; however, histologic examination of the interferon-treated tumour sites in Salvin's study (1975) revealed substantial infiltration by mononuclear cells.

It is quite remarkable that the various nonantiviral properties of interferon preparations are similar, if not identical to, the various biologic properties that have been described for lymphokines (Pick *et al.*, 1979; Waksman, 1979). Indeed, Salvin *et al.*, (1975) found that *in vivo* there was a close correlation between the conditions of sensitization that resulted in maximal production of lymphokines and interferon, and that both were associated with protection against aerosol challenge with a virulent strain of tuberculosis.

A number of studies from our own laboratory have demonstrated a variety of inflammatory mediators induced by viral infection of nonlymphoid cells. Although we initially thought these to represent yet additional properties of interferon, we were able to define conditions under which these activities were present in the absence of antiviral effects. In addition, we were able to define relationships between these factors and conventional lymphokines. These virus-induced products, which we defined as "cytokines" will be described in detail in the following section.

III THE CYTOKINES: LYMPHOKINE ACTIVITIES PRODUCED BY NONLYMPHOID CELLS

The first suggestion that a lymphokine-like activity could be generated by nonlymphoid cells came from the independent studies of Tubergen *et al.* (1972) and Papageorgiou *et al.* (1972) on MIF-like activity in established cell lines. Cell types studied included human and murine fibroblasts, HeLa cells, and hamster brain tumours. Subsequently, Papageorgiou *et al.* (1974) found that skin fibroblasts from immunodeficient patients could also give rise to MIF-like activity, providing additional evidence that the activities described were not due to lymphoid cell contamination.

These experiments raised the possibility that lymphokines or lymphokine-like substances can be produced by nonlymphoid cells. However, they were open to criticism on several grounds. There was, in some studies, a lack of control experiments to exclude the possibility that culture supernatants from nonlymphoid cells contained toxic substances capable of killing macrophages, thus inhibiting their migration. The viability of immobilized macrophages was not controlled and experiments were not extended beyond 24 h to check for resumption of migration. Moreover, since there was no sharply defined inducing stimulus, such as antigen in lymphoid cultures, a "non-stimulated" preparation was unavailable to serve as a reference control for macrophage migration. In addition, tests for other lymphokines were not performed, so that no information was available on the production of chemotactic factors and other mediators that augment rather than inhibit cellular responses and which could therefore not be simulated by toxic effects.

We began studies in this area with an attempt to define a system in which a well-defined stimulus triggered mediator production. We soon found that virus-infection of nonlymphoid cells led to the appearance of lymphokine-like activities. In one such study (Ward *et al.*, 1972) we demonstrated that allantoic fluids from chick embryos infected with Newcastle disease virus or mumps virus contain chemotactic activity for neutrophils and macrophages. Similar chemotactic activities were detected in supernatants from monkey kidney cell cultures infected with mumps virus. We found that these chemotactic factors were not associated with intact virus particles. Additional studies indicated that their production is a property of the infected cell rather than of the particular infecting virus. In these first experiments, the relationship between elaboration of interferon activity and leukotactic activity was not determined, but it was noted that the latter had a molecular weight of approximately 150 000, which is higher than that usually reported for interferon.

In a parallel study, our group also observed that supernatants from monkey kidney cell cultures infected with Newcastle disease virus or mumps virus contain MIF-like activity (Flanagan *et al.*, 1973). Again, it was shown that the mediator activity was not associated with virus particles. Viability studies on the guinea pig macrophages used as the target cells of the assay for MIF showed that the majority of the cells were viable and capable of resuming migration after incubation for 72 h. Both viability studies and the reversibility of migration inhibition showed that the results were not due to cytotoxic effects. The relationship between MIF-like activity and interferon was investigated and it was found that the appearance of MIF in supernatants of cultures infected with mumps virus preceded the appearance of interferon, while both MIF and interferon appeared simultaneously in supernatants from cultures infected with Newcastle disease virus. Viral inactivation studies showed that long periods of UV irradiation of Newcastle disease virus resulted in the loss of the capacity to stimulate MIF, while the ability to produce interferon was still present.

In addition to *in vitro* studies, *in vivo* experiments were also performed. Yoshida *et al* (1974) demonstrated that migration inhibitory activity can be detected in extracts of parotid glands from monkeys inoculated with mumps virus. Sephadex G 100 analysis of extracts from glands removed two and seven days after infection showed MIF-like activity in a peak corresponding to a molecular weight range of 45 000–65 000 as well as in a peak at approximately 12 000 daltons. Similar experiments on extracts from 23-d samples obtained from monkeys that had received a second dose of mumps virus 48 h prior to biopsy, showed a broad band of activity of lower molecular weight, in a range from 5000 to 30 000 daltons. These results suggest that the MIF activity induced *in vivo* is caused by multiple molecular species. The early activity, observed 2–7 d after primary infection is nonimmunologic, which is consistent with the finding that the MIF-like factors are comparable in size to those obtained following *in vitro* infection of nonlymphoid cells by mumps. The late activity, observed in 23 d extracts, has a considerably lower molecular weight, similar to classic MIF of primate origin and may be produced by antigen-stimulated lymphocytes in the parotid gland.

In the initial studies by our group, cytokine production by virus-infected nonlymphoid cells was first investigated with respect to infection by paramyxoviruses. For additional investigations, we then chose a DNA virus, SV_{40}, because of its specific interest as an oncogenic virus and because it is a poor interferon inducer (Bigazzi *et al.*, 1974). Supernatants from SV_{40}-infected and normal monkey kidney (AGMK) cells and from SV_{40}-transformed and normal human fibroblasts (WI–38) were tested for migration inhibition and chemotactic activities. Inhibition of macrophage migration was obtained with media obtained from cultures of SV_{40}-infected AGMK cells obtained 24, 48 and 72 h after infection, while no significant inhition was observed with media obtained after the third day of infection. When cells were observed for cytopathic effects, none were detected during the first two days of infection, but in the following days there was a steady increase in the percentage of affected cells. The MIF-like substance was not toxic for macrophages, as demonstrated by vital staining and the migration of these cells after continuous cultivation for more than 48 h. To rule out the possibility that residual virus in the fluids interfered with macrophage migration even in the absence of gross cytotoxicity, doses of virus identical to those used to infect AGMK cell cultures were added to cell-free medium, which was then centrifuged and UV-irradiated in the same manner as the supernatants from infected cultures. The resulting preparations were devoid of MIF-like activity. Supernatants from complete monolayers of normal and SV_{40}-transformed WI-38 cells also contained MIF-like activity. After fractionation by Sephadex G 100 chromatography, the MIF-like activity was found in two fractions, one corresponding to a molecular weight of 45 000 and the other to 12 000. "Classic" lymphocyte-derived MIF has also been localized in two fractions of similar molecular weight. In contrast to our previous studies with mumps and Newcastle disease virus, little or no chemotactic activity for neutrophils or macrophages was found in any of the media from SV_{40}-infected cell cultures.

Independently from our studies, similar observations were reported by two other groups of investigators. Hammond *et al.* (1974) observed that mouse fibroblasts transformed by SV_{40} virus elaborate a substance capable of inhibiting macrophage migration. In their experiments they noted that supernatants from cultures of SV_{40}-transformed 3T3 fibroblasts originally derived from BALB/c and Swiss mice contained an MIF-like activity. On the other hand, supernatants from normal 3T3 cells had little or no inhibitory activity. In contrast to the observations by other investigators, no relation was observed between release of MIF-like activity and cell division. Similarly to previous observations, the MIF was nondialysable, stable after heating at 56° or 80° for 30 min and eluted from Sephadex G 100 in the same molecular weight range as guinea pig lymphocyte-derived MIF.

Poste (1975) reported that supernatants from cultures of virus-transformed fibroblasts contained a substance inhibiting macrophage migration. The cells producing the MIF-like mediator were mouse fibroblasts transformed by SV_{40} and hamster fibroblasts transformed by polyoma or Rous sarcoma virus. In contrast, no significant MIF activity was detected in supernatants obtained from continuous cultures of untransformed mouse and hamster fibroblasts. In the same report it was also shown that a diverse range of human tumour cell lines, including HeLa, Detroit 562 and other cultures derived from osteogenic sarcoma, malignant melanoma, etc., released MIF activity in their culture media. No significant MIF activity was observed in supernatants from nontumour igenic human diploid cell strains, with the single exception of WI38 fibroblasts. Membrane ultrafiltration and Sephadex chromatography indicated that the MIF-like mediator had a molecular weight of approximately 25 000, was nondialysable, sensitive to chymotrypsin, more heat stable than lymphocyte-derived MIF and was inhibited by some trypsin inhibitors, DFP and EACA.

While most investigations summarized in this section have been concerned with the production of chemotactic factors and/or MIF by virus-infected cells, a recent study has shown that the DNA synthesis of HeLa cells was suppressed by culture fluids of cells infected with measles virus (Minagawa *et al.*, 1973; 1974). This suppression is induced by the viral infection but is not due to viral particles or envelope components. The product responsible for the suppression of host DNA synthesis is a nonvirion-associated, nondialysable heat stable protein, with no biological activities of measles virus. It was demonstrated in fractions of mol. wt 45 000, 20 000 and 3000. Cells damaged by the cytopathic effects of polio virus, vesicular stomatitis virus or Sindbis virus did not produce this substance, while, in addition to measles, mumps virus and Newcastle disease virus did. This substance when injected intravenously into mice decreased the number of circulating leukocytes in the blood of the injected animals.

In all the studies on production of cytokines by virus-infected and/or transformed nonlymphoid cells, normal cells were used as controls. Thus, we were able to observe that supernatants from complete monolayers of nontransformed WI-38 fibroblasts released MIF-like activity into the culture media (Bigazzi *et al.*, 1975). A comparison between macrophage migration inhibition obtained with supernatants of normal and SV_{40}-transformed WI-38 cells indicated that in the early stages of culture, transformed cells released more MIF-like substance than normal cells. However, it is possible that unavoidable differences in the metabolism of the two different cell types may have affected relative migration inhibitory activity in a nonspecific manner. Poste (1975) also detected MIF activity in supernatants of WI-38 fibroblasts tested on human lymphocytes, but observed no inhibition of migration with media from a variety of other nontumourigenic human diploid fibroblast strains. Similarly, no significant MIF activity was observed by Hammond *et al.* (1974) and Poste (1975) in supernatants from untransformed 3T3 mouse fibroblasts, hamster fibroblasts and primary cultures of mouse fibroblasts. This is in contrast with previous findings by Tubergen *et al.* (1972) and can be explained by differences in the sensitivity of the methods used to detect MIF or in the cell strains used in the experiments.

IV RELATION BETWEEN CYTOKINES AND LYMPHOKINES

In all the studies on the production of cytokines, attempts have been made to characterize the mediators produced and compare them to "classic" lymphokines. As could be expected, most of the information relates to MIF-like activities, which is not surprising since MIF is one of the best investigated lymphokines. In general, striking similarities between lymphocyte-derived and nonlymphoid cell-derived MIF have been reported.

Comparisons between lymphokines and cytokines have been usually made on the basis of molecular weight, resistance to heating and effects of dialysis. However, in our laboratory we have recently used other parameters to determine similarities between MIF derived from SV_{40}-infected monkey kidney cells and lymphocyte-derived MIF (Yoshida *et al.*, 1975a). The virus-derived MIF was absorbed on Sepharose bead columns conjugated with an antiserum prepared against lymphocyte-derived MIF (Yoshida *et al.*, 1975b) demonstrating that the two factors share at least some antigenic determinants. Moreover, SV_{40}-induced MIF was able to substitute for lymphocyte-derived MIF in an *in vivo* system involving the suppression of cutaneous manifestations of cellular immunity by intravenous injection of the lymphokine.

V RELATION BETWEEN CYTOKINES AND ANTIVIRAL INTERFERONS

Some of the criteria usually employed to define interferons are molecular weights in the range of 20 000–40 000 response to treatment with trypsin, heat and low pH and the property of species specificity. Unfortunately, these criteria are not uniformly met by all interferons and in fact, as is the case for MIF and other lymphokines, there is great heterogeneity of interferon with respect to molecular weight and other properties. The molecular weight of interferon induced in human skin fibroblasts by NDV is approximately 25 000–30 000, but values of human interferon induced by other viruses may reach up to 160 000 (Fantes, 1973). Monkey interferons induced in kidney cells by Sendai virus have a molecular weight of 13 000–25 000, while those induced by NDV have molecular weights of 35 000 and 160 000. Most mouse interferons range from 23 000 to 38 000, but several others have been described with molecular weights up to 100 000. If one compares these values of interferons with those of some cytokines, quite a few similarities become obvious. We found that chemotactic factors for neutrophils and macrophages detected in supernatants of mumps-infected monkey kidney cells had a molecular weight of 150 000, much higher than the values usually attributed to monkey interferons, but, as indicated above, a similar molecular weight has been reported for monkey interferon induced by NDV. Similarly, the molecular weights of MIF obtained after infection of monkey kidney cells with mumps, NDV and SV40 are 12 000 and 45 000–65 000, values not very dissimilar from those of monkey interferons. Mouse MIF has molecular weights of 25 000 and 35 000–50 000 similar to those of mouse interferons.

Thus, a distinction between interferons and the other cytokines based on molecular weight is rather unreliable. Lymphocyte-derived MIF is stable at 56°C and nonlymphoid cell-derived-MIF is stable at 80°C for 30 min; thus resistance to heat can be used to distinguish them from interferon. However, it has been pointed out that, even though most interferons are not very resistant to heat treatment, some are rather heat stable (Lockart, 1973).

Finally, the criterion of strict species specificity does not seem to hold true for all interferons (Lockart, 1973). However, cytokines seem to have no species specificity at all, since chemotactic factors obtained from chicken and monkey cells are active on rabbit macrophages and neutrophils, while MIF obtained from human, monkey and mouse cells is active on guinea pig macrophages and human lymphocytes.

Thus, because of the great heterogeneity of interferons, it is rather difficult to distinguish them from other cytokines. However, both resistance to heat treatment and lack of species specificity suggest that at least the MIF obtained from virus-infected or -transformed cells is different from interferons. This suggestion is further strengthened by some experiments performed by our group, aimed at determining the presence of MIF and interferon in supernatants from mumps and NDV-infected monkey kidney cells (Flanagan *et al.*, 1973). The presence of interferon was determined using monkey kidney cells infected with vesicular stomatitis virus. Mumps-infected monkey kidney cells released MIF in the supernatants 24 h after infection, when interferon was not detectable. After 48 h, more MIF was produced and interferon was also detected. On the other hand, in supernatants from NDV-infected monkey cells MIF production was detected at 48 h concomitantly with interferon. When NDV was inactivated by UV irradiation for 60 or 120 s, it was noted that the inactivated virus was still capable of inducing interferon, but not MIF production. Thus, in these experiments, a dissociation between production of interferon and MIF was noted, suggesting rather strongly that we are indeed dealing with two different types of mediators.

Finally, even though in our studies on production of MIF by SV_{40}-infected cells we did not assay for interferon production, the evidence available shows that SV_{40} is a very poor interferon inducer (Bigazzi *et al.*, 1975). There has only been one report showing that SV_{40}-infected African green monkey kidney cells produce an inhibitory substance, nondialysable, nonsedimentable, stable at pH 2·5 and inactivated by trypsin (Diderholm, 1963). This substance was defined as interferon, even though it was significantly more active in mouse cells than in monkey cells. Other studies have failed to show induction of interferon in monkey cells by several strains of SV_{40} (Plummer, 1963; Altstein, 1969). Recently Oxman (1973) has reported that SV_{40} did not induce measurable amounts of interferon either in monkey cells lytic virus-cell interaction) or in mouse cells (nonlytic virus-cell interaction). He concluded that at present there is no convincing evidence that SV_{40} induces formation of interferon, either during lytic or during transforming (nonlytic) virus-cell interactions.

The evidence summarized in this section suggests that, in spite of the great heterogeneity of interferons, even when defined in terms of classic antiviral activity, these mediators can be distinguished from other cytokines such as MIF. The distinction may not be easy because all these mediators are evaluated by their biological activities in *in vitro* systems and have not yet been satisfactorily purified and isolated. However, when the inevitable question arises of whether the viral-induced cytokines are just another aspect of an "interferon", one can now easily answer that at least MIF is distinguishable from interferon and that actually, because of the present state of the art, many of the various activities currently attributed to interferon in addition to its known ability to induce resistance to viral infections, might represent different products released by infected cells, similar to those we have defined in general as "cytokines".

VI POSSIBLE RELATIONSHIPS AMONG CYTOKINES, LYMPHOKINES AND INTERFERON

In this essay we have summarized experiments that demonstrate that interferon preparations have many nonantiviral properties that are similar to those of known lymphokines. Interferon may be induced not only by viral infection but also when the producing cell is a lymphoid cell, by mitogen or antigenic activation. This production appears to be macrophage dependent, as is the case for many conventional lymphokines.

The cytokines represent another set of mediators with properties identical to those of many lymphokines. At first glance it would seem then that the terms "interferon" and "cytokine" are synonymous. However, as described above, cytokine activities may be generated under conditions where antiviral interferon activity is limited or absent. Thus, we are faced with spectra of overlapping but non-identical activities. The issue is more than semantic because of the close physicochemical correspondence between lymphokines and cytokines. The best evidence for mediator identity here is for MIF, where as described above, (Yoshida *et al.*, 1975), we showed antigenic relationships between SV_{40}-induced, nonlymphoid cell-derived MIF, and antigen-induced lymphocyte-derived MIF.

Thus, all three classes of mediators may be related. In other words, the distinctions between lymphokines, cytokines and interferons may be more apparent than real. Direct proof of this contention, however, is difficult at the present state of the art. Studies on cytokines have focused on efferent lymphokine-like activities such as those affecting inflammatory cells. Studies of nonantiviral properties of interferons have usually, but not always, focused on afferent lymphokine-like activities such as those involved in immunoregulation. Although direct immunologic comparisons have been made between one cytokine and a corresponding lymphokine (MIF), no similar studies have been performed with respect to interferon associated non-antiviral activities and corresponding lymphokines. No systematic studies have been done on the reactivity of antilymphokine antibodies with interferon and vice versa. Now that great strides have been made in the purification of interferon, it should be possible to search for dissociation of biologic effects in different interferon fractions or preparations. To date, the only clear association is between antiviral activity and inhibition of cell proliferation (reviewed in Brouty-Boye, 1980).

These observations and considerations all suggest that there is an underlying phenomenon that we are all describing with the use of different labels. It may well be that there is a general capacity of many different cell types to produce mediators that regulate cell proliferation, cell migration and cellular activation. These may be related to similar factors that must play a crucial role in embryogenesis and development. Such mediators, during evolution, may have become adapted to serve the needs of host defence. To the factors described here, we can add nerve growth factor, epidermal growth factor, tumour angiogenesis factor and possibly many of the regulatory chalones. In this unifying view, the unique properties of each family of mediators may be confined to the kinds of cells that produce them, and the ways in which those cells are activated for their production. If this notion is correct, it would considerably simplify the present morass of multiple, apparently unrelated but biologically potent mediators and provide a hope for common pathways of action as well as similarities in function and overall molecular structure. It would indeed be a pleasant surprise if, in analogy to the case in modern physics, there turned out to be a set of universal biological "quarks" that formed the underlying basis for this vast panoply of mediators and activities that we are all struggling with. The term cytokine would then refer to the general set of these factors. Lymphokines would represent a subset induced in specific cells (lymphocytes) by certain specific (immunologic or mitogenic) stimuli. Interferon would refer to the antiviral mediator plus whatever additional functions that prove inseparable from that activity in molecules purified to homogeneity. On the basis of current evidence, the antiviral effects of interferon and the antiproliferative effects may be due to the same molecule. In contrast, all the effects on cell migration and cellular activation ascribed to interferon may turn out to be due to distinct cytokines.

Even if this general notion should prove incorrect, it suggests a number of fruitful experiments. For example, are there relationships between the antiviral activity, antiproliferative, and immunosuppressive activities of lymphokine preparations? Does purified interferon have migration inhibitory or chemotactic activities? Regardless of the outcome of these and other studies, the time seems ripe to search for underlying order amongst the mediators involved in host defence.

VII REFERENCES

Adelman, N. E., Hammond, M. E., Cohen, S. and Dvorak, H. (1979). *In* "The Biology of the Lymphokines" (Eds S. Cohen, E. Pick and J. J. Oppenheim), pp. 13–59. John Wiley, New York.

Altstein, A. D., Dodonova, N. N., Nadtochey, G. A. and Bykovski, A. F. (1969). *Arch. ges. Virusforsch.* **28**, 7–18.

Bigazzi, P. E. (1979). *In* "The Biology of the Lymphokines" (S. Cohen, E. Pick and J. J. Oppenheim, eds) pp. 243–258. J. Wiley, New York.

Bigazzi, P. E., Cohen, S., Ward, P. A. and Yoshida, T. (1974). *Fedn. Proc. Fedn. Am. Socs. exp. Biol.* **33**, 640.

Bigazzi, P. E., Yoshida, T., Ward, P. A. and Cohen, S. (1975). *Amer. J. Pathol.* **80**, 69–77.

Brouty-Boye, D. (1980). *Lymphokine Rep.* **1**, 99–112.

Brouty-Boye, D. and Zetter, B. R. (1980). *Science* **208**, 516–518.

De Maeyer, E., De Maeyer-Guignard, J. and Vandeputte, M. (1975). *Proc. natn. Acad. Sci. U.S.A.* **72**, 1753–1757.

Epstein, L. B. (1979). *In* "The Biology of the Lymphokines" (Eds. S. Cohen, E. Pick and J. J. Oppenheim) pp. 443–514. John Wiley, New York.

Fantes, K. H. (1973). *In* "Interferons and Interferon Inducers" (Ed. N. B. Finter) pp. 171–200. Elsevier, New York.

Flanagan, T. D., Yoshida, T. and Cohen, S. (1973). *Inf. Immunol.* **8**, 145–150.

Gresser, I. (1977). *In* "Cancer—A Comprehensive Treatise" (Ed. F. Becker), pp. 521–571. Plenum Press, New York.

Hammond, M. E., Roblin, R. O., Dvorak, A. M., Selvaggio, S. S., Black, P. H. and Dvorak, H. F. (1974). *Science* **185**, 955–957.

Isaacs, A. and Lindenmann, J. (1957). *Proc. R. Soc. Ser. B.* **147**, 258–267.

Isaacs, A., Lindenmann, J. and Valentine, R. C. (1957). *Proc. R. Soc. Ser. B.* **147**, 268–273.

Lockart, R. Z., Jr. (1973). *In* "Interferons and Interferon Inducers" (Ed. N. B. Finter) pp. 11–27. Elsevier, New York.

Minagawa, T., Nakaya, C. and Lida, H. (1974). *J. Virol.* **13**, 1118–1125.

Minagawa, T., Nakaya, C., Oguma, K. and Lida, H. (1973). *Japan. J. Microbiol.* **17**, 237–241.

Miorner, H., Landstrom, L. E., Larner, E., Larsson, I., Lundgren, E. and Strannegard, O. (1978). *Cell. Immunol.* **35**, 15–24.

Ngan, J., Lee, S. H. S. and Kind, L. S. (1976). *J. Immunol.* **117**, 1063–1066.

Oxman, M. N. (1973). *In* "Interferons and Interferon Inducers" (Ed. N. B. Finter) pp. 391–480. Elsevier, New York.

Papageorgiou, P. S., Henley, W. L. and Glade, P. R. (1972). *J. Immunol.* **108**, 494–504.

Papageorgiou, P. S. and Glade, P. R. (1974). *Cell. Immunol.* **12**, 326–330.

Pick, E., Cohen, S. and Oppenheim, J. J. (1979). *In* "The Biology of the Lymphokines" (Eds S. Cohen, E. Pick and J. J. Oppenheim) pp. 1–12. John Wiley, New York.

Plummer, G. (1963). *Br. J. exp. Pathol.* **44**, 58–65.

Poste, G. (1975). *Cancer Res.* **35**, 2558–2566.

Rosenstreich, D. L. and Wahl, S. M. (1979). *In* "The Biology of the Lymphokines" (Ed. S. Cohen, E. Pick and J. J. Oppenheim), pp. 210–242. John Wiley, New York.

Salvin, S. B., Nishio, J. and Shonnard, J. T. (1974). *Infect. Immunity.* **9**, 631–635.

Salvin, S. B., Ribi, E., Granger, D. L. and Youngner, J. S. (1975b). *J. Immunol.* **114**, 354–359.

Salvin, S. B., Youngner, J. S., Nishio, J. and Neta, R. (1975a). *J. natn. Cancer Inst.* **55**, 1233–1236.

Schultz, R. M. (1980). *Lymphokine Rep.* **1**, 63–98.

Schultz, R. M., Papamatheakis, J. D. and Chirigos, M. A. (1977). *Science* **197**, 674–676.

Sonnenfeld, G. (1980). *Lymphokine Rep.* **1**, 113–132.

Tubergen, D. G., Feldman, J. D., Pollock, E. M. and Lerner, R. A. (1972). *J. exp. Med.* **135**, 255–266.

Waksman, B. H. (1979). *In* "The Biology of the Lymphokines" (Eds S. Cohen, E. Pick and J. J. Oppenheim) pp. 585–616. John Wiley, New York.

Ward, P. A., Cohen, S. and Flanagan, T. D. (1972). *J. exp. Med.* **135**, 1095–1103.

Wheelock, E. F. (1965). *Science* **149**, 310–311.

Yaron, M., Yaron, I., Gurari-Rotman, D., Revel, M., Lindner, H. R. and Zor, U. (1977). *Nature, London* **267**, 457–459.

Yaron, M., Yaron, I., Smetana, O., Eylan, E. and Herzberg, M. (1976). *Arthritis Rheum.* **19**, 1315–1320.

Yoshida, T., Bigazzi, P. and Cohen, S. (1975a). *Proc. natn. Acad. Sci.* **72**, 1641–1644.

Yoshida, T., Bigazzi, P. E. and Cohen, S. (1975b). *J. Immunol.* **114**, 688–691.

Yoshida, T., Cohen, S., Bigazzi, P. E., Kuratsuji, T. and Amsden, A. (1975c). *Am. J. Pathol.* **81**, 389–400.

Yoshida, T., Flanagan, T. D., Genco, R. J. and Cohen, S. (1974). *Clin. Immunol. Immunopathol.* **2**, 472–480.
Yoshida, T., Sonozaki, H. and Cohen, S. (1973). *J. exp. Med.* **138**, 784–797.

Interferon Nomenclature: Report from the Committee on Interferon Nomenclature

COMMITTEE
William E. Stewart II (Chairman)*
J. Edwin Blalock (Galveston, TX)
Derek C. Burke (Coventry)
Charles Chany (Paris)
June K. Dunnick (Bethesda)
Ernesto Falcoff (Paris)
Robert M. Friedman (Bethesda)
George J. Galasso (Bethesda)
Wolfgang K. Joklik (Durham, NC)
Jan T. Vilček (New York)
Julius S. Youngner (Pittsburgh)
Kathryn C. Zoon (Bethesda)

Interest in interferons in recent years has become widespread; whereas, historically, interferons were primarily the concern of virologists, now immunologists, cell biologists, cancer biologists and others are also working with these substances. It has therefore become necessary to define as precisely as possible what is meant by "interferon," to classify the various interferons that have been discovered, and to devise a system for their orderly nomenclature. For this purpose an international group of scientists was assembled under the sponsorship of the National Institute of Allergy and Infectious Diseases and the World Health Organization-US National Centre on Interferon. This committee met at the National Institutes of Health in Bethesda, Maryland on March 7, 1980. The following is the unanimous report from this committee. It is hoped that workers in the various related fields and the editors of scientific journals publishing papers on interferon research will adopt this nomenclature, to avoid the proliferation of terms for the same substances and the indiscriminate naming of newly discovered factors.

The committee accepted the following definition for interferon: "To qualify

* Interferon Laboratories, Memorial Sloan-Kettering Cancer Center, 1275 York Avenue, New York 10021, USA

as an interferon a factor must be a protein which exerts virus non-specific, antiviral activity at least in homologous cells through cellular metabolic processes involving synthesis of both RNA and protein".

The preferred abbreviation for interferon is IFN. This abbreviation was chosen to eliminate the confusion of using the abbreviation IF, which could be confused with either the common abbreviation for initiation factor or the English word of that spelling. Each interferon will be identified according to animal of origin: e.g. human (Hu IFN); murine (Mu IFN); bovine (Bov IFN); rat (Rat IFN); chicken, porcine, feline, equine interferon, etc. However, it may be necessary in some cases to apply generic nomenclature: e.g. monkey = *Rhesus* interferon, etc.; fish = *Salmo* interferon, etc.; bat = *Taderida* interferon, etc.

Interferon will be classified into types on the basis of antigenic specificities. The type designations will be alpha (α), beta (β) and gamma (γ), corresponding to previous designations of leukocyte (Le), fibroblast (F), and Type II (immune) interferons, respectively. The old terminology of "leukocyte", "fibroblast" and "immune" interferons were, by committee consensus, abolished, as they clearly were misnomers: both leukocyte and fibroblasts can produce each of these two types of interferon, and "immune" interferons are often induced by mitogens rather than by immune recognition reactions. Also, the abbreviation "F" has often been used to designate either fibroblast or fast migrating interferons. Alpha and beta interferons are usually acid-stable and correspond to what have been called Type I IFNs; gamma interferons are usually acid-labile and correspond to what has been called Type II IFNs. If there are discovered to be classes of IFN which are not presently recognized, they should be designated sequentially IFN-delta, epsilon, etc. However, no IFN should be designated as to type until it has fulfilled the criteria for being so classified. Table I lists the new nomenclature for human and murine interferons and the corresponding designations which have been or are being employed. Interferon preparations may contain more

TABLE I Old and New Nomenclature for Human and Mouse Interferons

New nomenclature	Old nomenclature	
	Human	Mouse
IFN-α	Le (leukocyte), Type I, pH 2 stable foreign cell-induced	F (fast), C, Type I, pH 2 stable
IFN-β	F (fibroblast), Fi, Type I, pH 2 stable	S (slow), A, B, Type I, pH 2 stable
IFN-γ	IIF (immune) Type II, T, pH 2 labile, antigen-induced, mitogen-induced	immune (IIF), Type II, pH 2 labile, T, antigen-induced, mitogen-induced

than one type: for example, interferons derived from human lymphoblastoid cells and interferons from murine fibroblasts contain both IFN-α and IFN-β. These can be designated as to predominate type. Thus, the interferons presently employed in clinical trials are either HuIFN-α or HuIFN-β, or admixtures therefore.

The committee's recommendations apply at present only to human and murine IFNs, since there is insufficient information about IFNs from other animal species to allow differentiation into types. Workers using IFNs from other species are encouraged either to attempt preliminary classification based on antigenic homology with existing antisera specific for human or mouse alpha, beta or gamma IFNs, or to establish sequence homology with the known types of human and mouse interferons.

It is recognized that there may be size, charge, sequence and other heterogeneities within the designated IFN types. Currently, there is insufficient information available about the nature of these differences to allow designation of specific subtypes. Properly documented differences in molecular size appear to be useful parameters for differentiation until more stringent criteria (amino acid sequence, monoclonal antibodies) become available. Molecular weight designations may be indicated in parentheses, e.g. Hu IFN-α (18K) or Mu IFN-β (38K), or subtypes of IFNs based on specific amino acid sequence differences can be classified as Hu IFN-α_1, Hu IFN-α_2, etc.

Indication of interferon origin for those that behave antigenically similarly may also be helpful. Thus, interferon from human lymphoblastoid cells and interferon from human leukocytes are both classified antigenically as HuIFN-α, yet these interferons differ in certain amino acids. Therefore, the nomenclature HuIFN-α (Ly) or HuIFN-α (Le) may be used until such time as specific differences in amino acid loci have been established and subtype designations can be assigned. Also, it is now recognized that there are a number of forms of HuIFN-α that differ in certain amino acids; eventually these may be designated according to specific amino acids and their locations. Schemes for such designation of subtypes of each of the major IFN types will be developed at subsequent meetings of the Nomenclature Committee. The next meeting of the Committee will be held in April 1981. Suggestions and comments for consideration by the Committee should be forwarded to the Committee's Chairman.